AMERICAN JOURNAL of PUBLIC HEALTH
JUNE 2026
Issue 6

AJPH

A PUBLICATION OF THE
AMERICAN PUBLIC HEALTH ASSOCIATION

Climate Change and Health Inequities

- Hurricane Helene, Los Angeles Wildfires
- Extreme Heat in Arizona
- Greater Susceptibility in Marginalized Communities
- Policy, Structural Changes to Combat Climate Change Threats

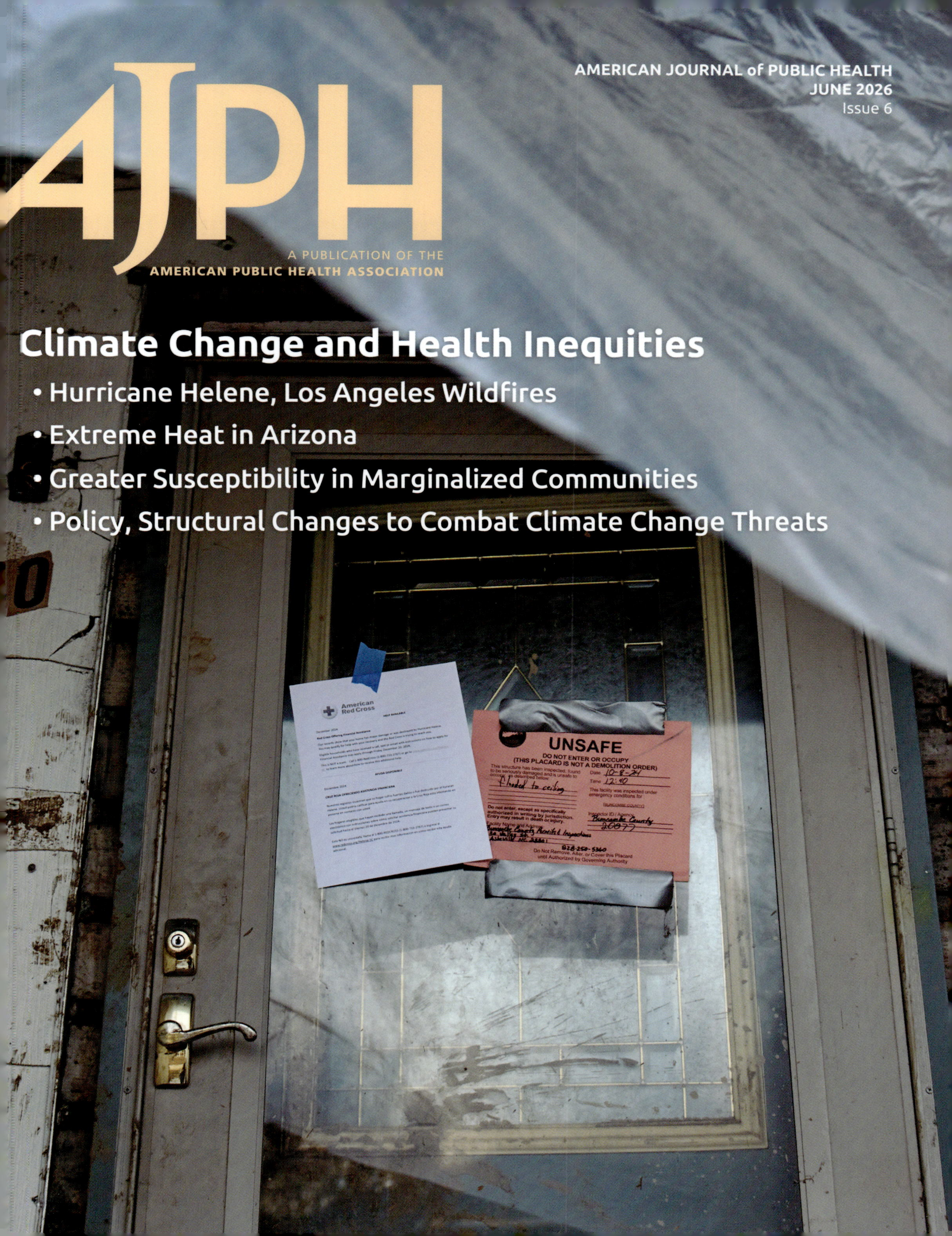

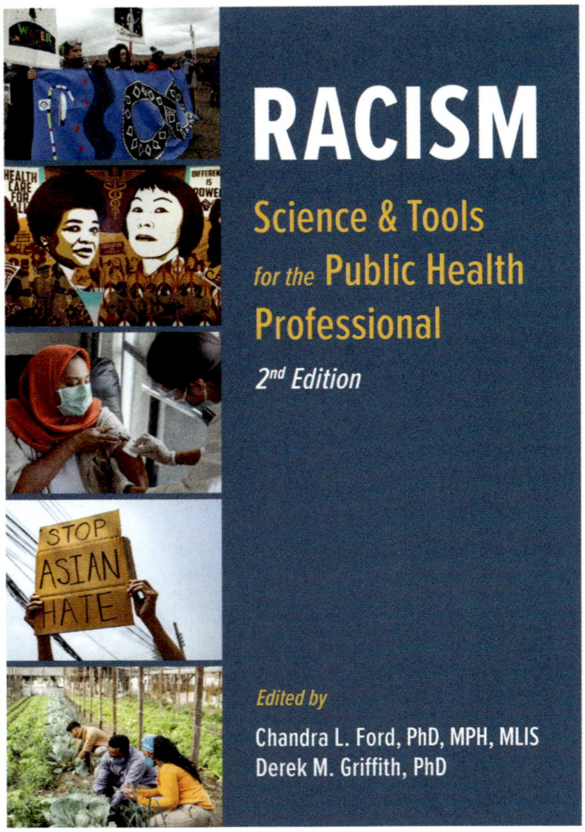

ISBN 978-0-87553-352-0, 600 PP., 2025, SOFTCOVER

Racism: Science and Tools for the Public Health Professional, 2nd edition

Chandra L. Ford, PhD, MPH, MLIS, and Derek M. Griffith, PhD

Racism: Science and Tools for the Public Health Professional, 2nd edition enables public health professionals to address the health impacts of racism. This vital title also responds to the watershed events of the past five years: the COVID-19 pandemic and its intersection with overt forms of racism across all socioecological levels, the 2020 murder of George Floyd by Minneapolis police and the unprecedented domestic and global movements toward racial justice that transpired, and other major global events.

APHABOOKSTORE.ORG

APHA PRESS

AN IMPRINT OF AMERICAN PUBLIC HEALTH ASSOCIATION

APHA
AMERICAN PUBLIC HEALTH ASSOCIATION
For science. For action. For health.

AJPH®, published monthly, is the official Journal of the American Public Health Association®, 800 I St NW, Washington, DC 20001-3710; (202) 777- APHA; TDD (202) 777-2500. APHA is a nongovernmental professional society founded in 1872, representing all disciplines and specialties in public health.

The *American Journal of Public Health*® (*AJPH*) (print ISSN: 0090-0036; electronic ISSN: 1541-0048), first published in 1911, is the official journal of the American Public Health Association® (APHA). The oldest and largest organization of public health professionals in the world, APHA represents approximately 30 000 members from more than 50 occupations of public health.

Submissions: Visit www.editorialmanager.com/ajph for online manuscript preparation and submission guidelines. Contributions of original unpublished research, social science analyses, scholarly essays, critical commentaries, departments, and letters to the editor are welcome. Questions? Write ajph.submissions@apha.org or call APHA at (202) 777-2469.

Print plus online subscriptions: Institutional price (print copy with online access) for a single institution and all authorized users, regardless of geographic location varies by size of organization; multiple campuses not permitted without special arrangement. To order, write apha.subscriptions@apha.org.

Online-only subscriptions: Institutional price for one US federal institution and its authorized users is $1,015–$1,510. To order, write apha.subscriptions@apha.org. For academic, non-US federal consortia, or multisite subscriptions, contact apha.subscriptions@apha.org or visit http://research.ebsco.com for pricing information.

Print-only subscriptions: Institutional price is US $970, $1,065 international.

Back print issues: A limited number of print issues are for sale. Single copies are US $80, $90 international (air delivery). Shipping and handling fees will apply; prepay only. To order, write apha.subscriptions@apha.org.

Reprints: For prices and ordering information on 50 or more reprints, check the Reprints section at www.ajph.org. To order smaller quantities of reprints (rush delivery), use the "Purchase Article" link on the article site itself.

Electronic access: Online articles more than 10 years old are available free for personal use at www.ajph.org. Recent articles are available through pay-per-view: single PDF article for $24, single issue access for 24 hours for $33, or entire site access for 24 hours for $38.

Postal information: Periodicals postage paid at Washington, DC, and additional mailing offices. Postmaster: Send address changes to American Journal of Public Health, 800 I St NW, Washington, DC 20001-3710.

Address changes: Send to AJPH, Membership Department (members) or AJPH Subscriptions (subscribers), APHA, 800 I St NW, Washington, DC 20001-3710. Or write to membership.mail@apha.org (members) or apha.subscriptions@apha.org (subscribers).

Advertising: For pricing and other information, see www.ajph.org. Please write to brian.selzer@apha.org or call (202) 777-2464 for other advertising opportunities. Ask about special exhibit packages and sponsorships. Acceptance of advertising by the *Journal* does not imply endorsement of products.

Indexes: Publications that index or abstract articles from *AJPH* include the following: Ageline, Assia (Applied Social Science Index and Abstracts), Biological Abstracts, Chemical Abstracts, CINAHL, Criminal Justice Abstracts, EMBASE, EMCare, Environmental Abstracts, e-psyche, ERIC, ETOH (Alcohol and Alcohol Problems Science Database), Excerpta Medica, Food Science and Technology, General Science Index, Grateful Med, Hospital Literature Index, Human Resources Abstracts, International Pharmaceutical Abstracts (IPA), Medline, Physical Education Index, Pollution Abstracts, Psychological Abstracts, PsychINFO, Safety Science Abstracts, Sage Family Studies Abstracts, Sage Human Resources Abstracts, Science Citation Index, SCOPUS, SIIC Data Bases, Social Work Research and Abstracts, and Statistical Reference Index (SRI)/LexisNexis.

AJPH
A PUBLICATION OF THE
AMERICAN PUBLIC HEALTH ASSOCIATION

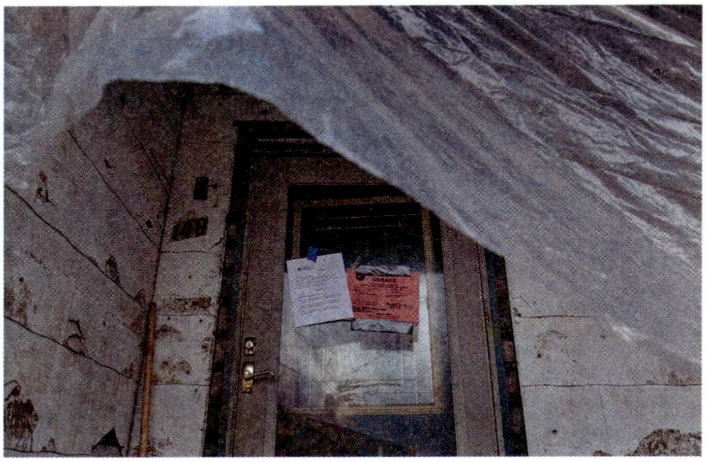

COVER: A sign from county officials declares Natalie Brigg's home is structurally unsafe, taped to her front door, in Swannanoa, NC, on Tuesday, December 3, 2024, after it was damaged during Hurricane Helene.

Cover concept and photo selection by Aleisha Kropf. Photo by AP Photo/Stephanie Scarbrough. Printed with permission.

APHA
AMERICAN PUBLIC HEALTH ASSOCIATION
For science. For action. For health.

Promoting public health research, policy, practice, and education is the *AJPH* mission. As we widen our scope to embrace global issues, we also sharpen our focus to support the needs of public health practitioners. We invite contributions of original unpublished research, opinion and commentary, and letters to the editor.

The *Journal* is printed on acid-free recycled paper.

AJPH June 2026, Vol. 116, No. 6

OPEN ACCESS — ONLINE ONLY — PODCAST — DATA SUPPLEMENT AVAILABLE

EDITOR'S CHOICE

741 Defending the Endangerment Finding: Science, Solidarity, and the Public Health Imperative
J. Balbus

OPINIONS, PRACTICE, & EDUCATION

EDITORIALS FROM THE ACADEMICS

743 Solutions-Oriented Science: Combating Fatalism Regarding Climate Change and Health
M. L. Ranney and J. B. Zimmerman

VACCINE ACCESS

746 The Need for Public Health Agencies to Collaborate and Innovate in an Era of Federal Instability: A View From the Northeast
I. Benowitz and E. S. Rosenberg

EDITORIALS

749 In Memoriam: William "Bill" Foege, Visionary Leader
J. W. Curran

751 What if They Had Asked Us? Recommendations From Former CDC Noninfectious Disease Leaders
K. Hacker, K. Remley, and G. M. Massetti

NOTES FROM THE FIELD

755 Enhancing Classification of Sexual Orientation and Gender Identity Information Among Suicide Decedents Reported in the National Violent Death Reporting System, 2003–2021
A. M. Anderson, L. D. Hughes, B. Rahman, and K. A. Clark

CLIMATE CHANGE/NATURAL DISASTERS

761 Climate Change and Health Inequities: Evidence and Action for Vulnerable Populations
T. Benmarhnia and N. Chartres

765 Climate Hazards and the Opioid Overdose Epidemic
J. A. Casey, B. D. L. Marshall, and M-A. Kioumourtzoglou

769 From Silos to Systems: Leveraging Technology to Bring Climate Health Insights to the Bedside and Back
A. Ramachandran, A. Teherani, and S. D. Weiser

772 Returning Public Health to the National Conversation on Climate Change
R. Sussman

775 Understudied Climate Change Attributes and Health Threats
A. Sapkota

777 Public Health Endangerment From Climate Change and Unnatural Disasters in the Anthropocene
M. Jerrett

RESEARCH & ANALYSIS

CLIMATE CHANGE/NATURAL DISASTERS

779 Mental Health Disparities From Climate Change: The Role of Housing Insecurity and LGBTQ+ Identity, California, 2023
E. Choa, D. Vlahov, and H. Poghosyan

790 Impact of the January 2025 Los Angeles Firestorm on People Experiencing Homelessness
E. M. Shannon, J. Chien, D. Paulazzo, G. Arreglo, B. F. Henwood, and R. Kuhn

798 Heat-Related Emergency Medical Services Activations in the United States, 2020–2024: Rates, Demographics, and Geographic Distribution
S. Saha, L. Jensen, C. S. Olsen, C. Gregor, B. Fisher, J. Balbus, A. Mataka, and N. C. Mann

806 Emergency Department Burden of Mental Health and Substance Misuse After Hurricane Helene: Insights From Rural Appalachia
M. M. Sugg, S. C. Ryan, A. Preaux, C. Quattro, B. Alexander-Eitzman, M. P. Thompson, A. Hege, and J. D. Runkle

810 Challenges and Opportunities in Estimating the Mortality Burden Related to Heat Exposure: Maricopa County, Arizona, 2019–2023
H. L. Leahy, A. Vaidyanathan, D. M. Hondula, M. Batchelor, N. M. Jarrett, R. N. Staab, R. Sunenshine, and A. P. Dale

OPEN-THEMED RESEARCH

814 Weakening Air Quality Standards Risks Reversing Health Gains
S. Tripathy

819 Abortion Bans and Maternal, Pregnancy-Related, and Pregnancy-Associated Mortality in 14 US States, 2016–2023: Estimated Impacts Amid Substantial Measurement Challenges
S. O. Bell, A. M. Franks, A. Ozinsky, S. Anjur-Dietrich, C. E. Margerison, E. A. Stuart, A. Feller, and A. Gemmill

829 Racial/Ethnic Differences in Homicides of Adult Women and the Role of Intimate Partner Violence: United States, 2018–2022
K. Forsberg, K. A. Fowler, B. H. Lyons, S. P. D. Jack, and J. M. Blair

841 Food Security by Racial and Ethnic Identity Among Lower-Income Adults
J. T. Denney

851 Trends in Meningococcal B Vaccine Uptake Among 16- and 17-Year-Old Adolescents in the United States: An Analysis of the National Immunization Survey–Teen, 2018–2023
N. P. Regmi, T. Xie, A. K. Ulrich, and N. E. Basta

855 Prevalence of Multiple Chronic Conditions Among US Adults, 2024
L. I. Black, A. E. Ng, B. Zablotsky, and B. W. Ward

859 Erratum In: "Science in Service: Reflections on the MacArthur 'Genius' Fellowship"

Defending the Endangerment Finding: Science, Solidarity, and the Public Health Imperative

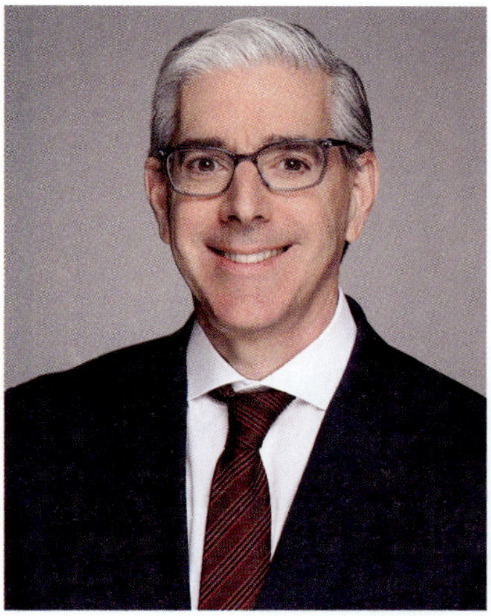

John Balbus, MD, MPH

The Clean Air Act has saved hundreds of thousands of lives, prevented millions of asthma attacks in children, and reduced millions of lost workdays—with benefits outweighing costs 30 to 1. How did it get so good?

SAVING LIVES THROUGH WISE REGULATION

One of the most powerful parts of the Clean Air Act (77 Stat. 392, Pub L No. 88–206; 1963) is known as the "Endangerment Finding." In a stroke of wisdom, the original authors of the Clean Air Act separated the question of whether an air pollutant harmed people from the question of how to respond. The determination of harm, which triggers the regulatory process, was to be based solely on scientific evidence of harm to human health or welfare.

That separation has worked well, enabling separate but effective processes to determine how to regulate air pollutants such as particulate matter and ozone and resulting in more than 230 000 lives saved by 2020. And the Endangerment Finding has never been questioned for any air pollutant. Until now.

In 2009, the Environmental Protection Agency (EPA) made an Endangerment Finding for the six most significant greenhouse gases, concluding with a reasonable degree of scientific certainty that those gases, by driving climate change, harmed human health and welfare. The finding followed a 2007 Supreme Court ruling in *Massachusetts v EPA* (549 US 497; 2007), which established that greenhouse gases met the Clean Air Act's definition of air pollution and compelled the EPA to act on a petition to regulate greenhouse gas emissions from transportation. It also followed the Second National Climate Assessment, published by the George W. Bush administration, which concluded that climate change threatened human health and welfare, primarily through increased heat, sea level rise, and worsening ozone pollution.

In 2009, I had been working on building awareness and understanding of the health impacts of climate change for 15 years. I had contributed to the health section of the Second National Climate Assessment and had the privilege of addressing the Senate Health, Education, Labor and Pensions Committee in 2008 as part of a panel discussing the health harms from climate change. My testimony focused on a study documenting that local public health officials were concerned about climate-related health impacts they were already observing but felt inadequately prepared to address them.

The ensuing 17 years massively strengthened the scientific evidence that climate change harms health. The Third National Climate Assessment, published in 2014, was the first to conclude that climate change was harming health in the United States now. The developing science of climate attribution has enabled us to identify a climate-specific toll on health: one landmark study found climate change responsible for 37% of heat-related deaths globally, and other major attribution studies have reached similarly sobering conclusions. And the evidence comes from our eyes, not just from scientific studies. Record-setting heat, such as the Northwest heat dome of 2021 and the massive increase in heat-related deaths in cities such as Phoenix, Arizona, since 2020, makes climate change's health impacts impossible to deny.

ENDANGERING LIVES THROUGH RECKLESS RESCISSION

And yet, that is exactly what the Trump administration is doing. On February 12,

AJPH June 2026, Vol. 116, No. 6

2026, the Trump EPA announced that it was rescinding the Endangerment Finding for greenhouse gases. In doing so, it is attempting to deny the reality that climate change is harming our health. The administration's attempt to justify the rescission with a scientific argument failed. The rescission is proceeding on questionable legal grounds, but the end result is the same: a denial that greenhouse gas pollution harms human health and welfare under the Clean Air Act and a decision to obstruct effective regulation.

This special *AJPH* issue is one of many critical contributions that not only reaffirm the Endangerment Finding but deepen our understanding of climate change's health impacts and strengthen our capacity to respond. Its articles illuminate new surveillance approaches for heat-related illness, the disproportionate burden borne by people experiencing homelessness, and the heightened risks facing people who misuse substances—shining a light in the darkness.

The *National Nature Assessment*, abandoned by the Trump administration but recently released in draft by its dedicated authors as the *Nature Record*, documents the mental health harms associated with contemplating climate change and the degradation of natural environments. The Fifth National Climate Assessment does as well. The scientific literature links greater mental distress to perceived political inaction on climate. I am not aware of a study specifically analyzing the mental health impacts of political malfeasance on climate change, but for those of us who care about this work, the rescission of the Endangerment Finding is more than an annoyance. It is psychological trauma.

THE PUBLIC HEALTH RESPONSE

How do we address this? How do we as public health professionals achieve our shared aim to improve and protect the health of all people, especially those suffering the greatest health burdens, and at the same time maintain our own resilience and motivation? This special issue is a piece of the solution. We must continue to study, to document, and to endeavor to prevent the health harms caused by climate change, even in the face of federal abandonment. Because the administration is relying on legal justifications, public health scientists can support the legal efforts to block and overturn the Endangerment Finding rescission. And lastly, we must acknowledge the trauma many of us are experiencing and support one another in community as we witness this political toxicity alongside accelerating climate change.

The desire for clean, healthy air for our children and our children's children unites us. The bipartisan wisdom of the Clean Air Act empowers us to achieve that desire. In the face of denialism, we have a responsibility to foster hope. The public health community must stand together in defense of that wisdom and ensure that political leaders who care about the nation's health have the best tools available to fight health-harming pollution. AJPH

DOI: https://doi.org/10.2105/AJPH.2026.308548

Solutions-Oriented Science: Combating Fatalism Regarding Climate Change and Health

Megan L. Ranney, MD, MPH, and Julie B. Zimmerman, MS, PhD

ABOUT THE AUTHORS

Megan L. Ranney is the dean of the School of Public Health, C.-E. A. Winslow professor of public health (health policy), and professor of emergency medicine, Yale University, New Haven, CT. Julie B. Zimmerman is vice-provost of planetary solutions and Liliane and Christian Haub professor of chemical and environmental engineering and the environment, and deputy director for research at the Center for Green Chemistry and Green Engineering, Yale University.

See also Editorials From the Academics Collection, https://bit.ly/3NEdvrc

Conversations about the impact of climate change on health often begin with urgency and end with resignation. We often hear people assert that we know what to do, but that it's too complicated, that an individual is impotent against complex multi-institutional systems, or that there is not enough political or economic will.

We reject this fatalism. The intersection of climate and health is not only one of the most important challenges of our time; it is also one of the most promising areas for innovation and collaboration to benefit public and planetary health. We suggest three accessible actions.

FIRST, ADVANCE SCIENCE THAT INFORMS SOLUTIONS

We know a lot about the impact of a changing climate on human health.[1] The increasing frequency and severity of storms and floods leads to injury, infectious diseases, and death. Wildfires degrade air quality and exacerbate asthma, cardiovascular disease, and adverse perinatal outcomes. Droughts heighten risks of dehydration and heat stress while undermining sanitation and hygiene. Changing temperatures expand the geographic and temporal spread of vector-borne and water-borne diseases; they also shape human and animal migration, thereby contributing to shifting patterns of human- and vector-borne diseases. Patterns of violence, overdose, workplace injury, mental illness, and more, are also well-established correlates of climate change.[2]

But measuring, monitoring, quantifying, and characterizing these harms is only the start.[3] The purpose of climate–health science is not simply to deepen understanding of risk, but to inform and empower solutions.

We need to understand how shifting ecological zones, changing species interactions, and altered environmental conditions change not just the spread of existing diseases, but also the emergence (and prevention) of new ones.[4] We must better quantify the economic and social costs of climate-related health impacts and disruptions. And we need more rigorous causal evaluations of the health consequences—both intended and unintended—of climate mitigation and adaptation strategies, ranging from urban greening to carbon capture.

Equally important for public health professionals and scientists is recognizing, and studying, the ways in which protecting environmental systems can benefit human health. The framework of planetary health[5] highlights how safeguarding ecosystems, mitigating climate change, and preserving biodiversity can simultaneously reduce disease, improve air and water quality, and strengthen conditions necessary for human well-being.

Each of these types of science can help inform decision-making by policymakers, community members, and the private sector—illuminating today's work and guiding what might happen in the future.

SECOND, BUILD CREATIVE PARTNERSHIPS FOR ACTION

Translating knowledge into impact necessitates collaboration not just among scientific disciplines but, equally importantly, between researchers and policymakers, community organizations, industry, and governments.[6] We recognize that this type of translation work is rarely incentivized or rewarded in academia, but simply discovering solutions is no longer adequate—action is needed, too.

For instance, after Hurricanes Ida and Maria, two communities recognized how storms, a fragile power grid, and limited health care access intersect. Nonprofit coalitions in Louisiana and Puerto Rico responded to the human health harms from these extreme weather events by developing and installing solar-powered microelectric grids in trusted community hubs. These hubs, ranging from churches to clinics, remain operational during storms and power outages, allowing residents to cool off during heat waves, safely store temperature-sensitive medications, access sanitary food and water, and find social support. The promise is that these microgrids will simultaneously support the short-term health needs of medically vulnerable populations, reduce greenhouse gas emissions, and eliminate reliance on polluting diesel generators during extreme weather events and power outages.

Together Louisiana has led the way in identifying solutions, partners, and funding for its Community Lighthouses program; in Puerto Rico, community health organizations, such as Casa Pueblo and the Clínica Esperanza/Hope Clinic, are leading. Both programs are supported by a variety of philanthropic and government entities as well as by partnerships with the private sector, such as local energy utilities.

The programs are not just built on trusted community relationships but are also being rigorously assessed to inform and scale subsequent work. Early assessments have shown that the solar initiative at Casa Pueblo mitigated immediate health risks while fostering a sense of security and well-being.[7] In Louisiana, the CDC Foundation and the National Academies of Science, Engineering, and Medicine are working to evaluate and improve the initiative's impact.[8] Duke University, with support from the Rockefeller Foundation, created Duke Cooling Communities, inspired by the Lighthouse work in Louisiana.[9] By linking clean energy deployment to health care access, centering community need and resources, and adding in rigorous academic evaluation, these models deliver climate mitigation, disaster resilience, and public health protection in one integrated solution.

These examples illustrate that most effective climate–health solutions often exist at the interface of constituencies. Multisectoral partnerships ensure that science-driven solutions have the political as well as financial means to continue, long after a research grant has been completed.

THIRD, LEAD BY EXAMPLE

At its best, public health has always connected knowledge to action. As academics and practitioners, we must lead by example, quickly creating and then translating evidence into interventions that improve health while protecting and restoring environmental systems.

We can lead by propagating a shared purpose and language behind climate–health solutions through shared principles. The climate–health intersection is not unique to red nor blue, rural nor urban, high- nor low-income people or geographies. In our experience, these putative barriers dissolve in the face of codevelopment of science or solutions based on a community-identified need. For example, our Yale Center for Climate Change and Health built deep partnerships both with large-city mayors across the globe to identify their cities' climate adaptation needs, and with rural political organizers who are concerned about mitigating environmental exposures. Neither of these partnerships fits into a typical ideological framework. Rather, they have pursued a purpose that is contextually relevant, locally appropriate, and scientifically as well as programmatically actionable. There are similar examples across the globe where our colleagues have taken the time to listen, thereby increasing the chances that their ideas will be trusted and used. We look forward to more such boundary-spanning work.

We also require new funding mechanisms. Although government funding remains paramount, philanthropic and private sector funds can help conduct and scale science more quickly. For instance, our Yale Planetary Solutions Catalyst Consortium is combining the university's interdisciplinary climate science expertise with the experience and leadership of corporate partners, creating a unique platform to identify and scale interventions that can touch the lives of millions in ways that our academic colleagues cannot do on their own. In the philanthropic world, we applaud the multifoundation collaborations that facilitated the creation, scaling, and evaluation of the solar-powered microgrids described here. Greater creativity is needed, and now is the time to pilot these innovative ways of closing well-recognized academic and practice gaps.

Finally, we urge tenacity. Climate and health challenges span years and systems, and we must collectively be courageous and relentless in insisting that our work truly delivers beneficial health outcomes while monitoring and mitigating unintended consequences.

The responsibility for solutions-oriented science has never been greater, nor the opportunity for impact more consequential. Fatalism is not an option. What matters most is that our efforts not just illuminate but ultimately advance and safeguard both human and planetary health. AJPH

CORRESPONDENCE

Correspondence should be sent to Megan L. Ranney, Yale School of Public Health, Laboratory of Epidemiology and Public Health, 60 College St, Suite #212, New Haven, CT 06510 (e-mail: megan.ranney@yale.edu). Reprints can be ordered at https://www.ajph.org by clicking the "Reprints" link.

PUBLICATION INFORMATION

Full Citation: Ranney ML, Zimmerman JB. Solutions-oriented science: combating fatalism regarding climate change and health. *Am J Public Health*. 2026;116(6):743–745.

Acceptance Date: March 13, 2026

DOI: https://doi.org/10.2105/AJPH.2026.308538

ORCID iD:
Julie B. Zimmerman https://orcid.org/0000-0002-5392-312X

CONTRIBUTORS

M. L. Ranney and J. B. Zimmerman contributed equally to the conceptualization and design of the work, drafting and revising the manuscript. M. L. Ranney approved the final version for publication.

ACKNOWLEDGMENTS

We thank the many colleagues, community partners, and practitioners whose work at the intersection of climate and health has informed the perspectives presented here.

CONFLICTS OF INTEREST

The authors declare no conflicts of interest.

REFERENCES

1. Crimmins A, Balbus J, Gamble JL, et al. The impacts of climate change on human health in the United States: a scientific assessment. US Global Change Research Program. 2016. Available at: https://www.healthandenvironment.org/docs/ImpactsClimageChangeHumanHealthUSGlobalChangeResearchProgramSmall2016.pdf. Accessed April 2, 2026.
2. Burke M, Wilson AJ, Avirmed T, et al. Understanding and addressing temperature impacts on mortality. National Bureau Of Economic Research. Published online October 2025. https://doi.org/10.3386/w34313
3. Mitchell D. Why we still don't know the mounting health risks of climate change. *Nature*. 2025; 637(8047):766–766. https://doi.org/10.1038/d41586-025-00149-5
4. Carlson CJ, Albery GF, Merow C, et al. Climate change increases cross-species viral transmission risk. *Nature*. 2022;607(7919):555–562. https://doi.org/10.1038/s41586-022-04788-w
5. Whitmee S, Haines A, Beyrer C, et al. Safeguarding human health in the Anthropocene epoch: report of The Rockefeller Foundation-Lancet Commission on planetary health. *Lancet*. 2015;386(10007): 1973–2028. https://doi.org/10.1016/S0140-6736(15)60901-1
6. Bowen SJ, Graham ID. From knowledge translation to engaged scholarship: promoting research relevance and utilization. *Arch Phys Med Rehabil*. 2013;94(1 suppl):S3–S8. https://doi.org/10.1016/j.apmr.2012.04.037
7. Madera SR, Varas-Díaz N, Padilla M, et al. Energy insecurity and health among older adults: chronic disease management and resilience strategies in rural Puerto Rico. *BMC Public Health*. 2026;26(1): 904. https://doi.org/10.1186/s12889-026-26558-3
8. O'Neill R. Community Lighthouses guide the way. CDC Foundation. March 28, 2025. Available at: https://www.cdcfoundation.org/blog/community-lighthouses-guide-way. Accessed March 6, 2026.
9. The Rockefeller Foundation. Turning community centers into heat-ready lifelines. Future-proofing health. Available at: https://www.rockefellerfoundation.org/future-proofing-health/turning-community-centers-into-heat-ready-lifelines. Accessed March 6, 2026.

The Need for Public Health Agencies to Collaborate and Innovate in an Era of Federal Instability: A View From the Northeast

Isaac Benowitz, MD, MPH, and Eli S. Rosenberg, PhD

ABOUT THE AUTHORS

Isaac Benowitz is with the Maine Center for Disease Control and Prevention, Augusta. Eli S. Rosenberg is with the New York State Department of Health, Albany.

See also *AJPH*'s Vaccine Access Collection, https://bit.ly/4l98J12

AJPH June 2026, Vol. 116, No. 6

The federal public health landscape shifted dramatically in 2025. Project 2025, the Make America Healthy Again agenda, and a vaccine-skeptic secretary of health and human services brought new public health priorities. Executive orders, grant rescissions, communications pauses, reductions in force, and budget proposals disrupted existing federal public health resources, questioning and dismantling foundational public health approaches that have saved countless lives.

Public health is a complex set of programs, services, and relationships bridging federal, state, local, and tribal public health agencies; health care; clinicians; payers; community organizations; academic institutions; and businesses. These and other groups work together to promote population health, protect vulnerable groups, and fill gaps in health care and other services. Public health agencies monitor infectious and chronic diseases and injuries at the population level, take action to control these conditions, and oversee environmental systems and health systems. They provide nutrition assistance, disease screening, immunizations, other clinical and prevention services, and health education and prepare for and respond to pandemics, earthquakes, mass casualty events, and other crises. The Northeast is home to more than 55 million people whose lives, education, and work overlap in a dense, highly interconnected region where health threats are not constrained by jurisdictional boundaries, enabling shared health priorities and opportunities for collective action.

State and local public health agencies rely heavily on federal infrastructure to deliver public health services.[1] The Centers for Disease Control and Prevention (CDC) operating budget, $11.6 billion in 2024, supports state and local public health agencies across the country and provides them with extensive resources: 80% of CDC's budget goes directly to these agencies. The other 20% goes into CDC programs that provide epidemiological, laboratory, and other technical and programmatic capacity and produce situational awareness, scientific guidance, health communications, and best practices across a wide range of public health areas, including emerging health threats such as Ebola, measles, and avian influenza.[2] These federal resources have become increasingly unstable through reductions in force, shuttered programs and laboratories, and disrupted funding. This collapse of federal capacity and the actions of leadership have eroded public trust in public health priorities and efforts.

Federal shifts and instability place populations at risk through diminished resources for state and local public health agencies, compounded by loss of federal scientific expertise and compromised public trust. Public health agencies must face this new hazard with the same planning and resilience they bring to natural disasters and disease outbreaks. They must build new strategies to ensure continuity of services that are less reliant on the hub-and-spoke model of public health that assumes federal capacity and guidance and involves replicating similar capacity in every state instead of leveraging interjurisdictional interdependence. Vaccine distribution, laboratory testing, emergency preparedness, communicable disease surveillance and response, chronic disease and injury surveillance and prevention, and other operations remain core priorities even if federal capacity and support shift abruptly. Public health agencies must also continue to work with the CDC and other federal government agencies and prepare for the federal government to resume more robust capacity and stability in the future.

By banding together, regional and other multistate groups can forge new ways to address these challenges. During past emergencies such as the

COVID-19 pandemic, northeastern states worked together to align economic policies and share resources.[3] Starting in early 2025, several state and large city public health agencies in the northeastern United States began meeting more often, building on a tradition of collaboration, to share information about disruptions and priorities and to develop shared approaches to support the continuity of services destabilized by reduced support from the federal government. The Northeast Public Health Collaborative (the Collaborative) emerged from these early conversations to strengthen existing relationships, increase support, and promote interdependence across public health agencies.[4]

In recent months, public health agencies have navigated numerous challenges in parallel, from federal agencies revising vaccine guidance and discontinuing treatment guidelines to disinformation on vaccines, autism, and gender. The Collaborative brings together public health agency staff across multiple subject areas to meet more regularly in a time of crisis to address shared leadership priorities. Key areas include communications, legal, preparedness, laboratory, workforce issues, immunizations, communicable diseases, and health care–associated infections. Workgroups share information and best practices and explore ways to integrate services across jurisdictions to ensure consistency and interoperability and take advantage of efficiencies of scale. Such efforts can increase the availability of data, strengthen the availability of services, promote trust through consistency, and support public health and population resilience.

The Collaborative has already started to bear fruit, strengthening an environment for the free exchange of ideas and helping public health agencies issue joint policy initiatives and shared communications. These include guidance for COVID-19, hepatitis B, and child and adolescent vaccine recommendations based on medical society guidelines; revised health care worker exclusion guidance after respiratory illnesses (building on the work of the now-disbanded Healthcare Infection Control Practices Advisory Committee); and several statements reaffirming vaccine science and guidance after changes in federal vaccine guidance.[5] Although the Collaborative has become adept at enabling public health agencies to collectively respond to crisis, shifting federal plans and the need to react in real time to mitigate harms present challenges in terms of planning ahead and preparing to fill larger gaps. Public health agencies share numerous operational needs that transcend political divides.

State and local public health agencies are stronger together, yet they cannot act alone: participation from other actors in the health ecosystem is essential. Other government agencies, health care systems, payers, professional societies, and community organizations share in these public health priorities and activities. Public health agencies can work with these other organizations to identify shared priorities for population health and explore opportunities for health care systems, payers, and others to take on greater roles. The recent AHIP (formerly America's Health Insurance Plans) statement that insurance plans will continue to cover routine vaccines is a strong first example.[6] The Collaborative is working with existing groups and other emerging health alliances throughout this ecosystem.

Public health remains essential even if national funding priorities shift, and new avenues are needed to fund the public health ecosystem. Collaboration and innovation can help to stabilize public health programs and services in the short term by using existing resources more efficiently; however, this will not address all deficits revealed by shifts in the federal government. Philanthropies can support infrastructure and create opportunities to support innovation, but they are unlikely to provide the long-term funding needed to sustained public health services. State and local policy initiatives can generate additional funding in some jurisdictions, and public health activities that generate revenue could help support other programs. Multistate approaches may lower costs, help to align strategies across borders, and ensure consistent services across jurisdictional lines.

The public health system is essential to a healthy population and society. Public health is always learning, evolving, and responding to crises. Collaboration across public health agencies in multiple jurisdictions, along with other organizations that play crucial roles in public health, is crucial in responding to any large-scale challenge. The current challenge is an attack on the established approach to setting and funding public health priorities at the national level. State and local agencies must and will continue to provide public health leadership and services, and regional collaboration is emerging as a crucial strategy for innovating and surviving in this emerging public health ecosystem. AJPH

CORRESPONDENCE

Correspondence should be sent to Isaac Benowitz, MD, MPH, Maine Center for Disease Control and Prevention, 286 Water St, 11 State House Station, Augusta, ME 04330 (e-mail: isaac.benowitz@maine.gov). Reprints can be ordered at https://www.ajph.org by clicking the "Reprints" link.

PUBLICATION INFORMATION

Full Citation: Benowitz I, Rosenberg ES. The need for public health agencies to collaborate and innovate in an era of federal instability: a view from the Northeast. *Am J Public Health*. 2026; 116(6):746–748.

Acceptance Date: March 12, 2026

DOI: https://doi.org/10.2105/AJPH.2026.308534

ORCID iD:
Isaac Benowitz https://orcid.org/0000-0002-1633-1985

CONTRIBUTORS

I. Benowitz drafted the work, and both authors revised it critically for important intellectual content. both authors made substantial contributions to the conception or design of the work.

ACKNOWLEDGMENTS

We thank Celia Quinn of the New York City Department of Health and Mental Hygiene for her substantial contributions to this work.

This article is part of an *AJPH* series on vaccine access and vaccination policies. Written by public health experts representing major organizations, these editorials tackle the current challenges the country faces in accessing vaccine care as governmental public health system undergoes transformation. Our intention is to spur thoughtful, scientifically sound ideas, rigorous research, and evidence-informed actions to protect population health. We welcome unsolicited editorials that are balanced, scientifically accurate, and self-reflective in examining one's own position to promote ongoing discussions as we work toward solutions that control vaccine-preventable diseases and support health and wellness nationally. See Ojikutu and Lau, available at: https://ajph.aphapublications.org/doi/epub/10.2105/AJPH.2026.308396

CONFLICTS OF INTEREST

The authors declare no conflicts of interest.

REFERENCES

1. National Association of County and City Health Officials. Local health department funding experiences. Available at: https://www.naccho.org/uploads/full-width-images/LHD-Funding-Experiences-UMN-V4-Mar-2025.pdf. Accessed March 11, 2026.
2. Centers for Diseases Control and Prevention. Putting prevention into public health practice. Available at: https://www.cdc.gov/washington/media/pdfs/2025/01/357075-B_Why-CDC_Factsheet.pdf. Accessed March 11, 2026.
3. Cohen R. Northeastern governors forge coalition to reopen their economies. Available at: https://csg-erc.org/northeastern-governors-forge-coalition-to-reopen-their-economies. Accessed March 11, 2026.
4. New York State Department of Health. Several northeastern states and America's largest city announce the Northeast Public Health Collaborative. Available at: https://www.health.ny.gov/press/releases/2025/2025-09-18_ph_collaborative.htm. Accessed March 11, 2026.
5. Dall C. Trump administration shuts down federal advisory committee on infection prevention. Available at: https://www.cidrap.umn.edu/healthcare-associated-infections/trump-administration-shuts-down-federal-advisory-committee. Accessed March 11, 2026.
6. AHIP. AHIP statement on vaccine coverage. Available at: https://www.ahip.org/news/press-releases/ahip-statement-on-vaccine-coverage. Accessed March 11, 2026.

In Memoriam: William "Bill" Foege, Visionary Leader

James W. Curran, MD, PhD

ABOUT THE AUTHOR

James W. Curran, MD, MPH, is a professor of epidemiology and dean emeritus of the Rollins School of Public Health, Atlanta, GA.

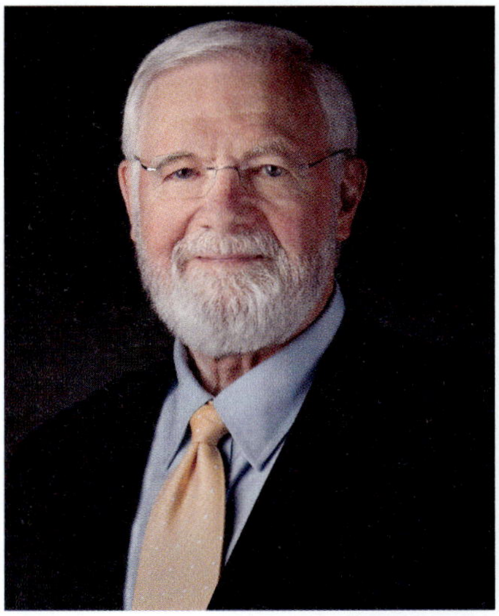

Portrait of William Foege, MD, MPH

An inspiring icon of public health, William Foege, MD, MPH, passed away peacefully on January 24, 2026, at home in Atlanta, Georgia, accompanied by Paula, his wife of more than six decades; their sons Robert and Michael; and their families. Foege (Bill to me) had served and led public health efforts on the ground, directing US and global institutions, and fostering collaborations throughout the world.

Born in Decorah, Iowa, in 1936, Foege graduated from Pacific Lutheran University (1957), University of Washington School of Medicine (1961), and Harvard School of Public Health (1965). Raised in a religious family with a father who was a minister, Foege was committed to social justice from the beginning and started his career as an Epidemic Intelligence Service officer at the Centers for Disease Control (CDC). He followed his public health training by moving with his family to Nigeria for work as a medical missionary. It was in 1965 in Nigeria that Foege first encountered smallpox, an infection that had no cure and cost the lives of at least 300 million people in the 20th century alone, while disfiguring countless millions more.[1] Though the effective smallpox vaccine was invented by Jenner in 1796, progress for control was very slow up until the World Health Organization (WHO) began a smallpox eradication campaign in 1959. The traditional approach, as with many infections, was mass vaccination, but this was very time-consuming, and vaccines were costly and scarce, so progress remained slow through the 1960s.

RING VACCINATION AND SMALLPOX ERADICATION

Working in eastern Nigeria from 1967 to 1968, Foege adapted a more efficient and effective approach. This approach of "ring vaccination" involved rapid identification and isolation of cases and priority vaccination of those who had been in contact with them. Next was vaccinating contacts of contacts and those gathering in public places. By advocating and utilizing this approach, smallpox was eradicated in West and Central Africa by 1970.[2] Foege was dispatched to India where implementation of this strategy led to smallpox eradication by 1975.[3] The last human case of smallpox was diagnosed in Somalia in 1978, and WHO declared smallpox to be eradicated throughout the world in 1980. Hundreds of millions of lives have been saved from smallpox since, and billions more people are spared the need to receive live smallpox vaccine. Foege recounted the lessons from these experiences in his first book, *House on Fire: The Fight to Eradicate Smallpox* (Berkeley, CA: University of California Press and Milbank Memorial Fund; 2011).

Smallpox remains the only infectious disease to be eradicated to date, and Foege's contributions have been widely recognized. Among the awards he received are the Mary Woodard Lasker Award for Public Service and Presidential Medal of Freedom (from President Barack Obama) in 2012, as well as the Presidential Citation, the highest honor from the American Public Health Association, of which he had served as president from 1986 to 1987.

CDC AND GLOBAL HEALTH

After the smallpox eradication campaign, the Foege family moved to Atlanta where Foege served as CDC director from 1977 to 1983 under both Presidents Carter and Reagan. His leadership there included CDC's role in the discovery and tracking of AIDS (where I first worked closely with him), and he guided CDC through those turbulent early years. Thanks to his visionary focus on prevention, Foege took CDC beyond infectious diseases to prevention of chronic diseases and disabilities, disabilities from environmental hazards, and intentional and nonintentional injuries. An inscription on a statue of Foege at the Sencer CDC Museum in Atlanta contains a quote from his farewell address to CDC:

> If the Centers for Disease Control is to maintain the reputation it now enjoys, it will be because in everything we do, behind everything we say as the basis for every program decision . . . we are willing to see faces.

Upon leaving CDC, Foege was approached by leaders of WHO, UNICEF, the United Nations Development Programme, the World Bank, and the Rockefeller Foundation to expand and coordinate global immunization for children, which then hovered at the 20% level. They sponsored him to form the Task Force for Child Survival (now the Task Force for Global Health). Foege led the Task Force from 1984 until 2000. This effort raised global immunization rates to 80% by the 1990s.

In 1986, President Carter approached Foege to become executive director of his newly formed Carter Center. Serving until 1992, Foege led the Carter Center to make global health an equal priority to its international peace initiatives. When President Carter, who died in 2024, was interviewed by the *New York Times* for Foege's eventual obituary, he stated:

> Bill Foege was a pre-eminent public health practitioner who dedicated his life to what he called science in the service of humanity. . . . He saved the lives of millions of people around the world.[4]

An example of Foege's wide influence in expanding public health collaborations involved working with pharmaceutical company CEOs on drug donation for neglected tropical diseases. The first, in 1987, involved the massive free donation for distribution of Mectizan (ivermectin) by Merck to control river blindness (onchocerciasis). The Task Force still manages the global distribution of this treatment and has expanded its "pharmacophilanthropy" partnerships to numerous other diseases and medications.

In 1997, I was reunited with Foege when he was recruited as Presidential Distinguished Professor of International Health at Rollins School of Public Health at Emory—a position he held as emeritus until his passing. In 1999, Bill Gates approached Foege for advice on programs to be taken by the new Bill and Melinda Gates Foundation. Foege helped guide the Foundation through 2009 on major global health initiatives, including public–private partnerships such as GAVI, the global vaccine alliance. In an October 2017 post for his "Gates Notes," describing how Foege had educated him and Melinda on global health, Gates wrote,

> There are few teachers as talented as Dr. Foege. As comfortable quoting Voltaire and Democritus as the latest *Lancet* article or World Health Organization report, Bill is always clear in his thinking about how much the world has accomplished in improving health as well as how much more we can do to alleviate human suffering.[5]

Foege's lecturing, writing, and advising continued to the end of his life. In addition to penning a fourth book, *Change Is Possible: Reflections on the History of Global Health* (Baltimore, MD: Johns Hopkins University Press; 2024), he helped develop "Becoming Better Ancestors: 9 Lessons to Change the World," a free virtual learning series that applies lessons learned in smallpox eradication to today's challenges. Foege's encyclopedic knowledge of past problems and successes in global health led to his singular optimistic forecast for the future despite current setbacks. According to Foege, future success requires science (finding the truth), collaborations, and commitment. He would say we are the ancestors for the future workers and the lives they will save.

Bill Foege was a man combining personal humility with far-reaching ambition for the health of others. He will be greatly missed, but his life is a living inspiration for all. AJPH

CORRESPONDENCE

Correspondence should be sent to James W. Curran, Rollins School of Public Health, Emory University, 1518 Clifton Rd NE, Atlanta, GA 30322 (e-mail: jcurran@emory.edu). Reprints can be ordered at https://www.ajph.org by clicking the "Reprints" link.

PUBLICATION INFORMATION

Full Citation: Curran JW. In Memoriam: William "Bill" Foege, visionary leader. *Am J Public Health*. 2026;116(6):749–750.

Acceptance Date: February 26, 2026.

DOI: https://doi.org/10.2105/AJPH.2026.308524

ORCID iD:
James W. Curran https://orcid.org/0000-0002-3268-9688

ACKNOWLEDGMENTS

Special thanks to Marian Moser Jones, PhD, for her help facilitating the publication process, as well as to the team at Johns Hopkins University Press for providing a portrait of William Foege.

CONFLICTS OF INTEREST

The author declares no conflicts of interest.

REFERENCES

1. Henderson DA. The eradication of smallpox—an overview of the past, present, and future. *Vaccine*. 2011;29(suppl 4):D7–D9. https://doi.org/10.1016/j.vaccine.2011.06.080.
2. Foege WH, Millar JD, Lane JM. Selective epidemiologic control in smallpox eradication. *Am J Epidemiol*. 1971;94(4):311–315. https://doi.org/10.1093/oxfordjournals.aje.a121325. PMID: 5110547.
3. Behbehani A. The smallpox story: life and death of an old disease. *Microbiol Rev*. 1983;47(4):455–509. https://doi.org/10.1128/mr.47.4.455-509.1983
4. Schneider K, Stolberg SG. William H. Foege, key figure in the eradication of smallpox, dies at 89. *New York Times*. January 24, 2026. Available at: https://www.nytimes.com/2026/01/24/us/william-h-foege-dead.html. Accessed April 7, 2026.
5. Gates B. Walking with a giant. *Gates Notes*. October 10, 2017. Available at: https://www.gatesnotes.com/Walking-with-a-Giant. Accessed April 7, 2026.

What if They Had Asked Us? Recommendations From Former CDC Noninfectious Disease Leaders

Karen Hacker, MD, MPH, Karen Remley, MD, MPH, MBA, and Greta M. Massetti, PhD

ABOUT THE AUTHORS

Karen Hacker is with Emory University, Rollins School of Public Health, Atlanta, GA, and is the former center director of the National Center for Chronic Disease Prevention and Health Promotion at Centers for Disease Control and Prevention (CDC). Karen Remley is with Emory University, Rollins School of Public Health, and is the former center director of the National Center for Birth Defects and Developmental Disabilities at CDC. Greta M. Massetti is with Georgia State University, School of Public Health, Atlanta, and is the former principal deputy of the National Center for Injury Prevention at CDC.

The past year has been tumultuous for the Centers for Disease Control and Prevention (CDC), marked by staff departures, reductions in force, leadership gaps, and uncertainty.[1] While attention has focused on infectious disease, particularly changes to the childhood vaccine schedule,[2] CDC's essential work on noninfectious diseases has been largely ignored. The agency's centers for chronic disease, injury, birth defects and developmental disabilities, and environmental health address the leading causes of morbidity and mortality in the United States, yet their future remains uncertain.

As former CDC leaders in chronic disease, birth defects, and injury prevention, we highlight the critical role of noninfectious disease programming and offer our recommendations to both the administration and the public health field for moving forward.

CDC's history with noninfectious diseases dates from the mid-1900s, as advances in treatment and vaccination[3] reduced infectious disease mortality and noninfectious conditions, such as heart disease, diabetes, cancer, suicide, and overdoses, became the largest killers of people in the United States.[4] Today, noninfectious causes drive nearly 90% of all deaths, with heart disease and cancer responsible for more than half. Among people in the United States aged younger than 44 years, injuries are the leading causes of death, due largely to drug overdoses and suicide.[4] Many of these deaths are preventable.

Prevention is the core function of noninfectious disease work at CDC. Over decades, historic impact was achieved via tobacco prevention,[5] cancer screening,[6] newborn screening, and injury prevention.[7] CDC awards more than 80% of appropriated funds to state, territorial, local, and tribal health departments and partner organizations to implement programs preventing diabetes, cancer, obesity, and overdoses and promoting nutrition and physical activity.

HOW CDC HAS PREVENTED NONINFECTIOUS DISEASE

To address noninfectious diseases, CDC leverages high-quality data to inform action, research, policies, and programs. Injury surveillance identified lack of seat belt use and impaired driving as preventable threats, directly informing laws and norms that reduced motor vehicle fatalities.[8–10] Tobacco surveillance and control supported smoke-free policies, excise taxes, and cessation efforts that drove historic declines in smoking and cancer. Data systems like the Behavioral Risk Factor Surveillance System (BRFSS) and the Youth Risk Behavior Surveillance System (YRBSS) guide prevention efforts related to nutrition, physical activity, and mental health, while overdose, maternal, infant, and birth defects surveillance have informed effective interventions such as opioid overdose prevention, folic acid fortification, and newborn screening. Together, these efforts underscore the critical public health role in noninfectious disease prevention.

IS THE ANSWER THE ADMINISTRATION FOR A HEALTHY AMERICA?

The current federal administration has advanced a narrow vision of CDC focused almost exclusively on infectious disease, asserting—without evidence—that noninfectious disease programs diluted the agency's pandemic response. In addition, they have argued that CDC should return to its core mission of infectious disease control and that

AJPH June 2026, Vol. 116, No. 6

noninfectious programming is redundant with other agencies. Toward this end, a new agency—the Administration for a Healthy America (AHA)—is being proposed. AHA would consolidate selected noninfectious disease functions of CDC, the Health Resources and Services Administration (HRSA), the Substance Abuse and Mental Health Services Administration (SAMHSA), and Office of the Assistant Secretary for Health (OASH).[11] The details of AHA are relatively opaque and largely come from the fiscal year 2026 and 2027 budget requests,[11] which propose to eliminate much of CDC's noninfectious programming and focus largely on individual health care approaches. There is no clarity about governance, preservation of statutory responsibilities, or protection of infrastructure necessary for accountability. In addition, this proposal, advanced without engagement of existing leadership or expertise, overlooks noninfectious disease monitoring (e.g., YRBSS, BRFSS, Pregnancy Risk Assessment Monitoring System) and population-based approaches to prevention (e.g., injury, diabetes, oral health, obesity programs). As a consequence, state and local health departments are left questioning the future of noninfectious disease efforts.

While AHA may have conceptual appeal, the absence of a coherent strategy that incorporates the population-based programming currently housed at CDC raises serious concerns. Prevention and health equity—the hallmarks of public health—were not prioritized. Proposed cuts and staffing reductions will leave some programs nominally funded but unable to operate. For example, Alzheimer's funding appears in the budget, but the program staff were eliminated in August of 2025. Other programs such as falls and drowning prevention and almost all of the chronic disease prevention programs (e.g., heart disease, diabetes, adolescent and school health, smoking, nutrition) and monitoring activities are nowhere to be found. Without explicit protections for this data, epidemiology, and prevention capacity, the reorganization risks undermining the federal infrastructure needed to address the nation's leading causes of death. At the time of this writing, the reorganization is not approved by Congress, lacks dedicated funding, and is stalled by litigation. If there is genuine interest in reorganizing federal noninfectious disease work, it should proceed through deliberate planning with public input. Alternatively, many goals could be achieved through clearer strategic coordination within existing structures.

WHAT IF THEY HAD ASKED US?

As public health leaders, we believe strongly that public health has an important role to play in preventing deaths and disability from noninfectious diseases. The clinical delivery system is ill-equipped to fill these population-based responsibilities at the national, state, or local level. But, while much has been successful in the noninfectious disease space, there are areas ripe for improvement across the Department of Health and Human Services (HHS). The time to consider this is now, for the current administration and for the field. Specific strategies for rebuilding will require feedback from a broad constituency. To begin, we offer a view of major issues that demand attention in efforts to reimagine a new public health, noninfectious disease infrastructure.

Coordinating Across the HHS

The fragmentation of efforts related to noninfectious diseases across HHS agencies has resulted in redundancy and confusion for the field. For example, numerous maternal and child health programs exist across HRSA, CDC, OASH, and Administration for Children and Families (ACF). This was particularly evident in the efforts to address maternal mortality (e.g., maternal mortality review committees at CDC and health care models funded at HRSA without a unified approach to the issue). Similarly, food and nutrition activities (regulation, safety, surveillance, and community programming) span US Department of Agriculture, Food and Drug Administration (FDA), CDC, and National Institutes of Health (NIH). Chronic disease programs (e.g., heart disease and diabetes) within CDC and across HHS (e.g., NIH, HRSA, and Centers for Medicare and Medicaid Services [CMS]) are not consistently or strategically aligned. Over time, legislative expansions without a shared strategic vision have produced these overlapping efforts without clear roles.

HHS should have responsibility for creating a unified strategic framework that aligns noninfectious disease programs across multiple agencies (i.e., CDC, HRSA, SAMHSA, OASH, NIH, FDA, and CMS), establishes roles and responsibilities, requires alignments of funding opportunities, and utilizes Healthy People 2030 measures to guide coordination.

Aligning Health Care and Public Health

The connections between public health prevention programs and the health care delivery system continue to be underdeveloped despite decades of attention.[12] Opportunities to align population-based public health prevention efforts such as the diabetes prevention program at CDC with new CMS care models (e.g., accountable care communities) and reimbursement strategies (e.g., ACCESS program, 1115 waivers) are missed opportunities. Data sharing between CDC and CMS remains challenging. Addressing these structural disconnects is essential to strengthening the federal role in noninfectious disease prevention. We must build a significant infrastructure bridge between CDC, FDA, NIH, and CMS such that data are shared, initiatives are strategically planned, and the public is clear about how agency responsibilities provide the most impact for the population.

Maintaining and Improving Data and Surveillance

CDC's public health data systems underpin the nation's ability to detect emerging threats, monitor trends, guide resource allocation, and evaluate progress. CDC should retain its role as the nation's lead agency for public health surveillance and epidemiological intelligence. At the same time, HHS must establish clearer policies for data integration across agencies. Decisions about where data reside, how systems are linked, the relationship with the private sector, and how data sets are shared should be intentional and transparent. For example, HRSA data on children's health should be combined with CDC data on childhood screening and developmental outcomes to create a more complete picture of child health. State, territorial, local, and tribal health departments partners must be actively engaged in planning, governance, and implementation as they are contributors and users of public health data.

Revaluation and Quality Improvement

Progress toward health outcomes should be regularly reviewed, reported transparently to the public, and adjusted accordingly using a formal, data-driven process. Here metrics like Healthy People 2030 are critical and will provide insight into current operations and future considerations. Part of reevaluation efforts includes recognizing when interventions previously implemented by one agency can transition to another. For example, the evolution of community health workers from CDC-supported pilots to CMS-reimbursable services illustrates how this transition can be managed effectively. These decisions should be based on disease burden, equity, effectiveness, reimbursement pathways, and state and local capacity.

Reorganization

The question of reorganization looms large. If HHS pursues reorganization, it should do so through a transparent process that engages Congress; state, territorial, local, and tribal health departments and other critical partners; and the public. There are naturally aligned functions across agencies that merit examination both across agencies and within agencies. Examples where reorganization could be considered include work on substance use, mental health, and suicide prevention across CDC and SAMHSA; child abuse and neglect efforts across CDC and ACF; maternal and child health activities across CDC, ACF, and HRSA; and chronic disease programs addressing shared risk factors like heart disease and diabetes within CDC and across NIH, HRSA, and CMS. Ultimately, reorganization could reduce administrative burden and enable states and localities greater flexibility to respond to local needs.

CHALLENGES

The current system has evolved over time. Line items in HHS agency budgets abound, add to the confusion of fragmented roles and responsibilities, and do not optimize outcomes. The aforementioned actions will take considerable effort and will require legislative support and financial realignment. Perhaps the greatest challenge is obtaining consensus from the myriad of interested parties across private and public sectors. The support for special interest groups, the public's attention to specific issues, and ofttimes competing agency agendas have led to the current situation. We must create a unified and compelling vision for the future of noninfectious disease interventions, and we urge the field to come together in this effort. Abrupt restructuring without safeguards risks disproportionately affecting communities already experiencing higher burdens of chronic disease, injury, and maternal and child health disparities.

Public health's role in preventing noninfectious disease is long and successful. Past achievements were not accidental; they were the result of deliberate choices based on data to prioritize prevention, build state and local capacity, and align science with policy. The leading causes of death and disability in the United States are overwhelmingly noninfectious, preventable, and shaped by social, environmental, and behavioral conditions that fall squarely within the purview of public health. Weakening the federal infrastructure that supports surveillance, prevention, and data-to-action programming risks reversing decades of progress.

At a time when noninfectious conditions account for nearly 90% of US deaths, retreating from prevention will represent a fundamental misalignment between federal priorities and the nation's health needs. As a nation, preserving the federal government's core strengths in data, science, and state partnership while improving coordination, reducing duplication, and modernizing systems offers a pragmatic alternative to dismantling capacity. The choices made now will determine the future of America's health for years to come. AJPH

CORRESPONDENCE

Correspondence should be sent to Karen Hacker, MD, MPH, Emory University, Rollins School of Public Health, Department of Health Policy and Management, 1518 Clifton Rd, Atlanta, GA 30322 (e-mail: karen.hacker@emory.edu). Reprints can be ordered at https://www.ajph.org by clicking the "Reprints" link.

PUBLICATION INFORMATION

Full Citation: Hacker K, Remley K, Massetti GM. What if they had asked us? Recommendations from former CDC noninfectious disease leaders. *Am J Public Health*. 2026;116(6):751–754.

Acceptance Date: March 13, 2026.

DOI: https://doi.org/10.2105/AJPH.2026.308544

ORCID iDs:

Karen Hacker https://orcid.org/0000-0001-6654-2935

Greta M. Massetti https://orcid.org/0000-0002-3813-9839

CONTRIBUTORS

All authors made substantial contributions to the conceptualization and writing of the work. K. Hacker led the writing of the commentary. All authors were also involved in drafting and revising the article and gave final approval of the version to be published.

CONFLICTS OF INTEREST

No authors have any conflicts of interest from funding or affiliation-related activities.

REFERENCES

1. Dietrich DR, von Aulock S, Bal-Price A, et al. The alarming consequences of workforce reductions at the FDA, EPA, NIH and CDC in the United States. *Arch Toxicol*. 2025;99(6):2239–2241. https://doi.org/10.1007/s00204-025-04065-5
2. Daval CJR, Kesselheim AS. The Advisory Committee on Immunization Practices—legal roles, challenges, and guardrails. *JAMA*. 2025;334(8):669–671. https://doi.org/10.1001/jama.2025.11400
3. Centers for Disease Control and Prevention. Ten great public health achievements—United States, 1900–1999. *MMWR Morb Mortal Wkly Rep*. 1999;48(12):241–243.
4. Centers for Disease Control and Prevention. WISQARS Leading Causes of Death Visualization Tool. Available at: https://wisqars.cdc.gov/lcd/?o=LCD&y1=2023&y2=2023&ct=10&cc=ALL&g=00&s=0&r=0&ry=2&e=0&ar=lcd1age&at=groups&ag=lcd1age&a1=0&a2=199. Accessed January 31, 2026.
5. Farrelly MC, Chaloupka FJ, Berg CJ, et al. Taking stock of tobacco control program and policy science and impact in the United States. *J Addict Behav Ther*. 2017;1(2):8.
6. Ma ZQ, Richardson LC. Cancer screening prevalence and associated factors among US adults. *Prev Chronic Dis*. 2022;19:E22. https://doi.org/10.5888/pcd19.220063
7. Chhatwal J, Mueller PP, Chen Q, et al. Estimated reductions in opioid overdose deaths with sustainment of public health interventions in 4 US states. *JAMA Netw Open*. 2023;6(6):e2314925. https://doi.org/10.1001/jamanetworkopen.2023.14925
8. Bergen G, Peterson C, Ederer D, et al. Vital signs: health burden and medical costs of nonfatal injuries to motor vehicle occupants—United States, 2012. *MMWR Morb Mortal Wkly Rep*. 2014;63(40):894–900.
9. Jewett A, Shults RA, Banerjee T, Bergen G. Alcohol-impaired driving among adults—United States, 2012. *MMWR Morb Mortal Wkly Rep*. 2015;64(30):814–817. https://doi.org/10.15585/mmwr.mm6430a2
10. Centers for Disease Control and Prevention. Motor-vehicle safety: a 20th century public health achievement [erratum in *MMWR Morb Mortal Wkly Rep*. 1999;48(22):473]. *MMWR Morb Mortal Wkly Rep*. 1999;48(18):369–374.
11. Department of Health and Human Services. Administration for a Healthy America. 2025. Available at: https://www.hhs.gov/sites/default/files/fy-2026-aha-cj.pdf. Accessed August 28, 2025.
12. Institute of Medicine. *Primary Care and Public Health: Exploring Integration to Improve Population Health*. 2012. Available at: https://www.nationalacademies.org/read/13381/chapter/1#ii. Accessed March 31, 2026.

Enhancing Classification of Sexual Orientation and Gender Identity Information Among Suicide Decedents Reported in the National Violent Death Reporting System, 2003–2021

Avery M. Anderson, PhD, MS, Landon D. Hughes, PhD, Banapsha Rahman, MPH, and Kirsty A. Clark, PhD, MPH

We developed and refined a systematic keyword search process to flag sexual orientation and gender identity indicators in National Violent Death Reporting System suicide narratives (2003–2021). Applying this process to 298 662 records resulted in 2580 records being flagged for review; 1221 (47%) were classified as sexually or gender minoritized (SGM), increasing the sample of identified SGM decedents by 32%. Our findings highlight persistent failures in accurate surveillance, limiting understanding of SGM suicide mortality. Narrative review methods enhance SGM identification and can improve evidence-based suicide prevention and public health policy. (*Am J Public Health*. 2026;116(6):755–760. https://doi.org/10.2105/AJPH.2026.308460)

AJPH June 2026, Vol. 116, No. 6

The National Violent Death Reporting System (NVDRS) is a state-based surveillance system containing suicide data from multisource primary documents, including death certificates, law enforcement reports, and coroner and medical examiner reports. Investigative findings include information collected from decedents' family and friends, personal communications (e.g., text messages, e-mails), and suicide notes. Trained abstractors code relevant death details and create two one-paragraph narratives from law enforcement and coroner or medical examiner reports describing events leading to the suicide.

INTERVENTION AND IMPLEMENTATION

The NVDRS began data collection in 2003 with six states and has since expanded to all 50 states, the District of Columbia, and Puerto Rico. The system added codes for sexual orientation and transgender status in 2013 and codes for same-sex partnerships in 2015. Between January 2003 and December 2021, data include 348 112 suicide records, with 3805 precoded by abstractors as sexually or gender minoritized (SGM). The overarching goal of our methodological study was twofold: (1) to develop a systematic keyword search process capable of capturing narrative indicators of sexual orientation and gender identity (SOGI) information and (2) to apply that search process with subsequent researcher reviews to improve classification of SGM suicide decedents from 2013 to 2021 and expand identification of SGM individuals before SOGI fields were added (2003–2012).

PLACE, TIME, AND PERSONS

In the current study, we analyzed NVDRS records lacking precoded SGM status (n = 344 307). We excluded records without sufficient substantive detail for SOGI identification (e.g., narratives of less than 15 words [n = 15 001] and records with "unknown" circumstances around death [n = 25 302]) and murder–suicide cases (n = 5342), yielding a narrative review sample of 298 662 records. Precoded SGM records were considered ground truth in this study because the abstractors had access to original, comprehensive documentation surrounding each suicide.

PURPOSE

Despite evidence of disproportionate suicide risk among SGM populations,[1–4]

national surveillance systems remain unequipped to reliably identify SGM suicide decedents.[5,6] Existing limitations in accurate SOGI data collection (e.g., bias, structural misclassification, and inconsistent ascertainment)[5] hinder understanding of structural and social contributors to SGM suicide mortality and impede responsive, evidence-based suicide prevention strategies. Earlier work established procedures to systematically classify death records by SGM status via narratives in national suicide surveillance systems[7,8]; however, analyses extend only through 2017, and previous procedures lacked contemporary enhancements such as adding "nonbinary" as a search term. Thus, our aim here is to adapt and expand previous suicide death record narrative review approaches[7,8] toward enhanced systematic classification of SGM decedents.

EVALUATION AND ADVERSE EFFECTS

We adapted and expanded earlier approaches[7,8] to systematically flag and subsequently review law enforcement and coroner or medical examiner narratives for SOGI information through multistep development of a keyword search process (Figure 1). Initially, the narratives were cleaned by removing descriptors that might break a string (e.g., "his new boyfriend" with "new" removed) and standardizing lowercase text. Then we began building the search process by updating a previously developed[7] list of search terms with greater inclusiveness of keywords and phrases. To do so, we examined precoded SGM narratives to identify phrases not previously captured (e.g., "not a woman/man," "identifying as a woman/man"). Next, the team brainstormed missing verbiage and added terms accordingly (e.g., "nonbinary," "sex change").

We applied the refined keyword list to precoded SGM narratives to assess the case detection ability of new terms. Iterative team reviews, prioritizing conceptual relevance and case detection, informed removal of terms with very low case detection (less than 15%) and minimal relevance after team consensus (e.g., "partner" detected in less than 2% of cases). To enhance detection of same-sex partnerships, we incorporated pronoun imputation by cross referencing phrases such as "victim's boyfriend" in the narratives with the decedent's

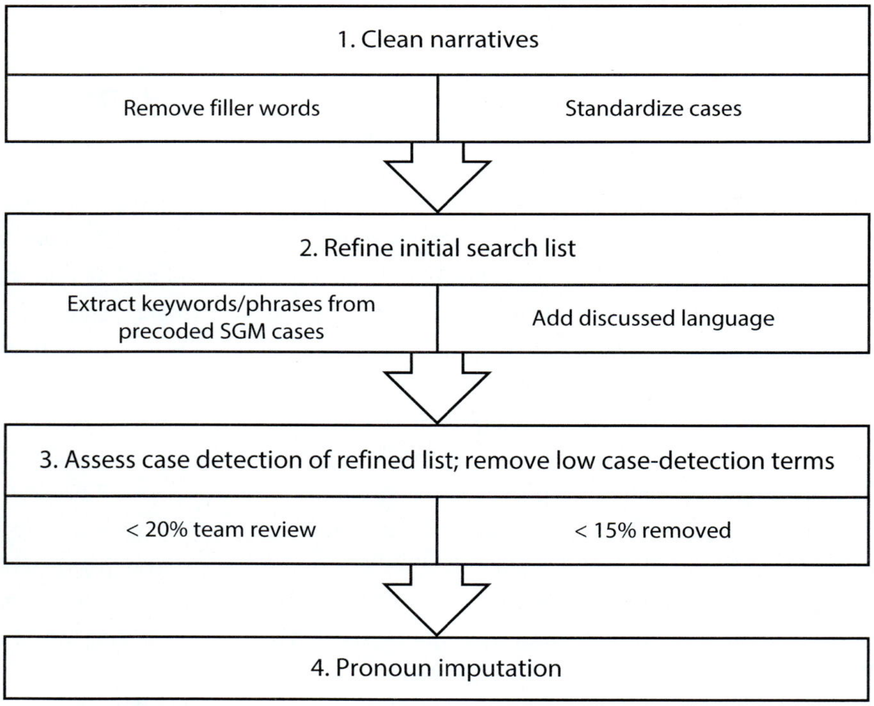

FIGURE 1— Process Model for Preparing and Building the Keyword Search

Note. SGM = sexually or gender minoritized.

recorded sex. After multiple refinement cycles, the final components of the keyword search process were documented for transparency and replicability (see Appendix A, available as a supplement to the online version of this article at http://www.ajph.org). Applying this keyword search process to 298 662 records resulted in 2580 (0.9%) records being flagged for SGM classification, as described subsequently.

Once flagged by the keyword search process, every flagged record that included SGM-relevant keywords was reviewed by the research team to ultimately classify SGM status through systematic coding and consensus. The team reviewed all 2580 flagged cases for SGM classification using a detailed coding guide delineating specific examples of coding procedures (see Appendix B, available as a supplement to the online version of this article at http://www.ajph.org). Because narratives are abstractor derived rather than self-reported, postmortem SGM classification is constrained by informants' and abstractors' perceptions, bias, and interpretation as well as by their ability to accurately identify and report SOGI information.

As such, we classified records according to plausibility on the basis of the available narrative information. Consistent with previous research,[7] we classified decedents as plausibly SGM if they met any of the following criteria:

1. they self-identified as SGM,
2. they were perceived as SGM,
3. they were perceived as exploring or questioning their sexuality or gender identity,
4. they described SOGI as a concern,
5. they were thought to experience gender dysphoria or were socially (e.g., changing name or pronouns) or medically (e.g., hormone therapy) transitioning, or
6. they were in a relationship with, attracted to, or consensually sexually active with a same-sex partner.

The coding guide (Appendix B) distinguished sexual orientation from gender identity, each with detailed criteria and examples. Thus, records were coded dichotomously (yes or no) on two dimensions: (1) plausibly sexually minoritized (e.g., lesbian, gay, bisexual) and (2) plausibly gender minoritized (e.g., transgender, nonbinary, gender questioning).

Three research team members independently coded the same random 10% subsample of records (n = 258) to assess consistent application of the coding guide. Given the emotionally taxing nature of reviewing suicide narratives,[9] coders engaged in reflective journaling for five to 10 minutes after each coding session. Subsequent meetings involved processing reflections and providing peer support before reviewing codes. During these meetings, coded records were reviewed, differences were adjudicated, and the coding guide was further refined. Then coders independently coded a new 10% subsample of records. Interrater reliability was 94% across coders, and the team collectively adjudicated the discrepant 6%. The remaining 80% of records were split evenly among coders to complete. Each coder could flag records for guaranteed discussion, and flagged records (n = 87; 3%) were coded by consensus.

In summary, 1221 (47%) of the 2580 records flagged and reviewed were classified as plausibly SGM by the research team. Thus, the total sample of SGM suicide decedents in the 2003 to 2021 NVDRS data was 5026, as compared with the precoded 3805, reflecting a 32% increase in SGM status ascertainment. Furthermore, the sample consisted of 4241 (84%) sexually minoritized decedents and 913 (18%) gender minoritized decedents. Sample demographic characteristics are described in Table 1. Among the 4241 plausibly sexually minoritized decedents, 1635 (39%) were female, 2478 (58%) were male, and 128 (3%) were unknown. Gender minoritized decedents cannot be accurately described by assigned sex because of highly variable gender and sex reporting across primary source documents.[5]

Our study advances previous efforts to address a critical gap in national mortality surveillance data. Using a multistep systematic approach, we identified an additional 1221 decedents as plausibly SGM in the 2003 to 2021 NVDRS suicide data. This represents a 32% increase from existing precoded data. Although rigorous methodological approaches to existing NVDRS data are strongly encouraged, they do not overcome all inherent limitations of existing SOGI information. The high false-positive rate (53%) in our enhanced keyword search process underscores challenges in relying on narrative-based classification. Likewise, even improved classification relies on incomplete and biased data, and our findings should not be interpreted as reflecting the true proportion of SGM suicide decedents.[10]

SUSTAINABILITY

Sustainability is not relevant in the context of this research.

PUBLIC HEALTH SIGNIFICANCE

This study offers one of the most comprehensive and systematically derived approaches to identifying SGM people

TABLE 1— Demographic Characteristics and Precipitating Suicide Circumstances by SGM Status: United States, National Violent Death Reporting System, 2003–2021

	Plausibly SGM Classified (n = 5026), No. (%)	Non–SGM Classified (n = 343 086), No. (%)
Age, y		
10–17	481 (9.57)	11 269 (3.28)
18–24	980 (19.50)	35 839 (10.45)
25–34	1 241 (24.69)	57 096 (16.64)
35–44	835 (16.61)	57 625 (16.80)
45–54	776 (15.44)	65 339 (19.04)
55–64	481 (9.57)	55 730 (16.24)
≥ 65	231 (4.60)	60 121 (17.52)
Missing/unknown	1 (0.02)	67 (0.02)
Sex		
Female	1 635 (32.53)	73 398 (21.39)
Male	2 478 (49.30)	269 626 (78.59)
Missing/unknown[a]	913 (18.17)	62 (0.02)
Race/ethnicity		
Hispanic/Latinx	508 (10.11)	22 706 (6.62)
Non-Hispanic American Indian/Alaska Native	66 (1.31)	4 458 (1.30)
Non-Hispanic Asian/Pacific Islander	137 (2.73)	8 116 (2.37)
Non-Hispanic Black	397 (7.90)	22 890 (6.67)
Non-Hispanic White	3 806 (75.73)	279 865 (81.57)
Another race, multiracial, or unspecified	111 (2.21)	4 662 (1.36)
Missing	1 (0.02)	389 (0.11)
Marital status		
Married, civil union, domestic partnership	948 (18.86)	110 618 (32.24)
Never married, single	3 366 (66.97)	127 392 (37.13)
Divorced, separated, widowed	659 (13.11)	101 220 (29.50)
Unknown	3 (0.06)	280 (0.08)
Missing	50 (0.99)	3 576 (1.04)
Education		
High school/equivalent or less	2 218 (44.13)	165 399 (48.21)
Some college or associate degree	1 286 (25.59)	67 922 (19.80)
Bachelor's degree	648 (12.89)	33 844 (9.86)
Any graduate school or higher	332 (6.61)	16 762 (4.89)
Unknown	480 (9.55)	53 653 (15.64)
Missing	62 (1.23)	5 506 (1.60)
Census region		
Northeast	803 (15.98)	52 481 (15.30)
Midwest	1 128 (22.44)	75 162 (21.91)
South	1 402 (27.89)	129 028 (37.61)
West	1 668 (33.19)	84 499 (24.63)
Missing	25 (0.50)	1 916 (0.56)

Continued

AJPH June 2026, Vol. 116, No. 6

TABLE 1— Continued

	Plausibly SGM Classified (n = 5026), No. (%)	Non-SGM Classified (n = 343 086), No. (%)
Precipitating circumstances		
Family relationship problem	614 (12.22)	23 340 (6.80)
Intimate partner problem	1 975 (39.30)	84 349 (24.59)
Other relationship problem (e.g., friend, associate)	350 (6.96)	12 284 (3.58
History of mental health or substance use treatment	2 283 (45.42)	108 472 (31.62)
History of suicide attempt	1 668 (33.19)	58 765 (17.13)
Current mental health problem	2 893 (57.56)	143 847 (41.93)
Current physical health problem	715 (14.23)	64 714 (18.86)
Recent suicide of family member or friend	169 (3.36)	6 580 (1.92)

Note. SGM = sexually or gender minoritized. All χ^2 *P* values are <.001.
[a]Missing data in plausibly SGM classified are largely due to gender minority status.

who die by suicide and provides a foundation for future public health research. Our work also demonstrates the feasibility of employing supplemental and scalable methods for improved SGM identification in suicide mortality data when structural barriers to SOGI data collection are being enforced. Indeed, the federal administration has executed intentional data erasures resulting in loss of critical public health information, including SOGI data.[11] Specifically, mentions of gender identity or transgender status have disappeared from the 2025 NVDRS codebook and data request forms, making the narrative identification approach outlined here potentially the only way to identify transgender people in forthcoming NVDRS data releases. As data erasure and invisibility persist, it is imperative that public health professionals and researchers demand data integrity, apply rigorous methods, and communicate existing data limitations across all dissemination channels.

Our findings underscore the urgent need for national surveillance systems to incorporate specific, precoded SOGI fields and strengthen abstractor training to ensure accurate identification of decedent identities. They should also motivate researchers to leverage innovative methods such as large language models to further enhance precise classification of SGM populations. AJPH

ABOUT THE AUTHORS

Avery M. Anderson is with the College of Nursing, University of Colorado Anschutz Medical Campus, Aurora. Landon D. Hughes is with the Department of Population Medicine, Harvard Pilgrim Health Care Institute, and Harvard Medical School, Boston, MA. Banapsha Rahman is with the Department of Population Medicine, Harvard Pilgrim Health Care Institute. Kirsty A. Clark is with the Department of Medicine, Health, and Society and the Department of Psychology and Human Development, Vanderbilt University, Nashville, TN.

CORRESPONDENCE

Correspondence should be sent to Avery M. Anderson, PhD, MS, College of Nursing, Mailstop C288, 13120 E 19th Ave, Aurora, CO 80045 (e-mail: avery.m.anderson@cuanschutz.edu). Reprints can be ordered at https://www.ajph.org by clicking the "Reprints" link.

PUBLICATION INFORMATION

Full Citation: Anderson AM, Hughes LD, Rahman B, Clark KA. Enhancing classification of sexual orientation and gender identity information among suicide decedents reported in the National Violent Death Reporting System, 2003–2021. *Am J Public Health*. 2026;116(6):755–760.

Acceptance Date: February 2, 2026.

DOI: https://doi.org/10.2105/AJPH.2026.308460

ORCID iDs:
Avery M. Anderson https://orcid.org/0000-0002-2751-1316

Kirsty A. Clark https://orcid.org/0000-0002-9626-8460

CONTRIBUTORS

A. M. Anderson drafted the initial article. A. M. Anderson and L. D. Hughes conceptualized the study and led data coding, analysis, and interpretation. L. D. Hughes developed the algorithm. B. Rahman participated in data coding and contributed to interpretation of findings. K. A. Clark provided the foundational study design, participated in data coding, contributed to interpretation of findings, and oversaw all aspects of the study. All of the authors contributed critical revisions to the article.

CONFLICTS OF INTEREST

Landon D. Hughes received grants from the American Public Health Association during the conduct of this study. Kirsty A. Clark reports receiving grants from the National Institutes of Health outside the submitted work. The other authors report no conflicts of interest.

HUMAN PARTICIPANT PROTECTION

This study involved a secondary analysis of deidentified data and did not meet the regulatory definition of human participant research.

REFERENCES

1. di Giacomo E, Krausz M, Colmegna F, Aspesi F, Clerici M. Estimating the risk of attempted suicide among sexual minority youths: a systematic review and meta-analysis. *JAMA Pediatr*. 2018; 172(12):1145–1152. https://doi.org/10.1001/jamapediatrics.2018.2731

2. Becerra-Culqui TA, Liu Y, Nash R, et al. Mental health of transgender and gender nonconforming youth compared with their peers. *Pediatrics.* 2018 May;141(5):e20173845 2018;141(5): e20173845. https://doi.org/10.1542/peds.2017-3845
3. Zachry CE, O'Brien RP, Clark KA, Ding ML, Blosnich JR. Mortality among sexual and gender minority populations: A systematic review. *PLoS One.* 2025;20(2):e0307688. https://doi.org/10.1371/journal.pone.0307688
4. Wolford-Clevenger C, Cannon CJ, Flores LY, Smith PN, Stuart GL. Suicide risk among transgender people: a prevalent problem in critical need of empirical and theoretical research. *Violence Gend.* 2017;4(3):69–72. https://doi.org/10.1089/vio.2017.0006
5. Clark KA, Blosnich JR. Limitations of sexual orientation and gender identity information as reported in the National Violent Death Reporting System. *LGBT Health.* 2024;11(3):173–177. https://doi.org/10.1089/lgbt.2022.0297
6. Haas AP, Lane AD, Blosnich JR, Butcher BA, Mortali MG. Collecting sexual orientation and gender identity information at death. *Am J Public Health.* 2019;109(2):255–259. https://doi.org/10.2105/AJPH.2018.304829
7. Clark KA, Cochran SD, Maiolatesi AJ, Pachankis JE. Prevalence of bullying among youth classified as LGBTQ who died by suicide as reported in the National Violent Death Reporting System, 2003-2017. *JAMA Pediatr.* 2020;174(12):1211–1213. https://doi.org/10.1001/jamapediatrics.2020.0940
8. Lyons BH, Walters ML, Jack SPD, Petrosky E, Blair JM, Ivey-Stephenson AZ. Suicides among lesbian and gay male individuals: findings from the National Violent Death Reporting System. *Am J Prev Med.* 2019;56(4):512–521. https://doi.org/10.1016/j.amepre.2018.11.012
9. Dasgupta N. Ghost in the machine: the emotional gravity of conducting mortality research. *Am J Public Health.* 2021;111(suppl 2):S80–S81. https://doi.org/10.2105/AJPH.2021.306378
10. Clark KA, Blosnich JR, Haas AP, Cochran SD. Estimate of lesbian, gay, bisexual, and transgender youth suicide is inflated. *J Adolesc Health.* 2019;64(6):810. https://doi.org/10.1016/j.jadohealth.2019.03.003
11. Shendruk A, Rampell C. How Trump is reshaping reality by hiding data. Available at: https://www.washingtonpost.com/opinions/interactive/2025/government-data-trump-deletion. Accessed March 11, 2026.

Climate Change and Health Inequities: Evidence and Action for Vulnerable Populations

Tarik Benmarhnia, PhD, and Nicholas Chartres, PhD, MHum Nutr

ABOUT THE AUTHORS

Tarik Benmarhnia is with Scripps Institution of Oceanography, University of California, San Diego, and the UC Center for Climate Health and Equity, University of California, San Francisco. Nicholas Chartres is with the School of Pharmacy, Faculty of Medicine & Health, University of Sydney, Sydney, Australia, and the UCSF Center to End Corporate Harm, University of California, San Francisco. Both authors are AJPH *associate editors.*

See also Climate Change/Natural Disasters, pp. 765–813.

Climate change has become politicized to such a degree that scientists and public health professionals have had to develop multiple creative strategies to continue their work. Yet the impacts of climate change on population health are far from invisible and are recognized as some of the most pressing public health and environmental justice challenges of our time. These challenges are manifested through increasingly frequent and severe weather events, chronic environmental stressors, and profound health inequities that disproportionately affect marginalized communities.[1] People in these marginalized communities have contributed least to greenhouse gas emissions yet have the fewest resources to adapt to their consequences.

As the climate and health research community faces mounting political pressure, it becomes even more critical to document health impacts, identify who is most affected and why, determine which adaptation strategies are effective and equitable, and urgently communicate and disseminate these findings to the public, health professionals, journalists, and policymakers.

PATHWAYS LINKING CLIMATE HAZARDS TO HEALTH OUTCOMES

The health consequences of climate change operate through multiple interconnected pathways that intensify existing climate threats, result in new threats, and reduce threats. First, climate change exacerbates existing environmental and weather-related determinants of health by increasing the intensity and frequency of exposures such as extreme heat events. Second, climate change creates unprecedented situations, particularly through compounded climate events that occur when multiple hazards overlap in time or space.[2] For instance, co-occurring wildfires and extreme heat events are becoming more frequent in California, and recovery time between successive events continues to shrink, leaving populations with less

Continued on page 762...

HISTORY CORNER

18 YEARS AGO

Climate Change: The Public Health Response

Several well-established principles point to a vigorous, proactive public health approach to climate change. One such principle is prevention. . . . There are clear analogies in the approach to climate change. Primary prevention corresponds to mitigation—efforts to slow, stabilize, or reverse climate change by reducing greenhouse gas emissions. Secondary and tertiary prevention corresponds to adaptation—efforts to anticipate and prepare for the effects of climate change, and thereby to reduce the associated health burden. Mitigation efforts will occur mainly in sectors other than health, such as energy, transportation, and architecture (although the health sciences can contribute useful information regarding the choice of safe, healthful technologies). Adaptation efforts, on the other hand, correspond closely to conventional medical and public health practices. This set of practices is collectively known as *public health preparedness.*

From *AJPH*, March 2008, pp. 435, 437.

24 YEARS AGO

Native Traditional Knowledge About Global Warming and Environmental Change

As far back as the 1970s, Alaska Native communities reported changes we now know to be time to recover and governments less time to adequately respond and prepare. Third, climate mitigation strategies offer opportunities to promote public health cobenefits. For example, reducing transportation emissions can promote active transportation, leading to increases in physical activity and decreases in exposure to traffic-related air pollutants.[3]

Climate change is fundamentally an environmental justice issue, characterized by what we term the "triple jeopardy" from differential exposure, susceptibility, and adaptive capacity. Differential exposure arises when some communities are systematically more exposed to climate-sensitive hazards (e.g., heat waves, floods) than are others. Differential susceptibility follows from the intersection of other determinants of health, such as occupation, discrimination, and food insecurity, with climate threats that increase the health burden among some subgroups. Differential adaptive capacity is caused by unequal resources to prepare for, respond to, and recover from climate-related effects across communities. A fourth dimension of environmental justice is differential evidence, whereby investigation and dissemination of evidence of harm or benefit to a community is lacking or suppressed. A first step to addressing an issue is to document it and make it visible.[4] Indeed, if this were not so important, current federal efforts to prevent these investigations and dissemination would not be so relentless.

CLIMATE-HEALTH BURDENS OF UNDERSTUDIED GROUPS

This *AJPH* issue's featured section responds to the urgent need for evidence by presenting research on understudied and marginalized populations that are inadequately represented in climate health research while also identifying challenges and opportunities in existing surveillance and prevention systems. The six articles featured here span diverse climate-sensitive exposures, from the highly visible disasters of Hurricane Helene and the 2025 Los Angeles wildfires to the less visible but equally deadly threat of extreme heat in Arizona, and these contributions document the complex pathways through which climate change threatens health and deepens existing inequities.

The first two articles in this featured section examine differential susceptibility. Choa et al. (p. 779) examine the intersection of housing insecurity and LGBTQ+ (lesbian, gay, bisexual, transgender, queer, questioning, asexual, intersex, and other nonheterosexual, noncisgender) identity as compounding factors in climate-related mental health effects. They found that bisexual and pansexual individuals and transgender and gender-expansive adults experienced higher risks of mental health burdens from climate events than did other adults.

Casey et al. (p. 765) provide a conceptual framework for understanding how climate hazards may exacerbate the opioid overdose epidemic through multiple interconnected pathways. These pathways include direct physiological effects (e.g., heat exposure increasing sedative effects of opioids), disruptions to medication access for those with opioid use disorder, trauma and stress from climate events, infrastructure damage affecting health care systems,

Continued on page 763...

HISTORY CORNER

associated with global warming, such as changing weather patterns, thinning ice, diseased and deformed wildlife, and changes in the look and taste of such subsistence foods as fish and meat. These early observations have been borne out by scientific research conducted in recent years. . . The Traditional Knowledge and Contaminants project uses a community-based model, which begins with local observations of environmental and health effects. These observations lead to community-driven research, assessment within the context of community-driven values, and finally, community-based conclusions and action. . . . The Traditional Knowledge and Contaminants Project database is composed of approximately 2000 entries from more than 400 participants representing 150 communities. It is updated at yearly regional meetings and as requested by individuals or communities at any time. . . . Traditional knowledge can provide scientists with more accurate and timely hypotheses to use in their search for the causes of declines in wildlife, saving time, money, effort, and undue delay in action. It can provide an early warning system for emergent biological or environmental trends and anomalies.

From *AJPH*, September 2002, pp. 1404, 1406.

and displacement leading to interruptions in treatment.

The next two articles examine the consequences of two events intensified by climate change and the triple jeopardy experienced by vulnerable populations. Shannon et al. (p. 790) provide critical insights into how people experiencing homelessness were affected by the January 2025 Los Angeles County firestorm. The authors conducted a survey and found that among 374 unhoused respondents, 76.5% reported life disruption or injury from the firestorm. Sugg et al. (p. 806) present findings on mental health and substance use emergency department utilization following Hurricane Helene in North Carolina. They found sustained increases in alcohol-related visits across all recovery periods, as well as increases in anxiety disorder visits, mood disorders during early recovery, and schizophrenia visits during short-term recovery.

An effective public health response to climate change requires robust surveillance systems capable of detecting health impacts in near real time and informing prevention strategies. Two articles in this collection demonstrate both the power and limitations of existing surveillance tools.

Saha et al. (p. 798) examine heat-related emergency medical services activations across the United States from 2020 to 2024. Among 79 077 804 emergency medical services activations during April through September, 261 687 (0.3%) were heat related. Activation rates were higher among older adults, males, African Americans, and Native Hawaiian/Pacific Islanders, as well as in rural counties and counties with worse socioeconomic and environmental conditions. Leahy et al. (p. 810) estimate that 3036 deaths (2019–2023) in Maricopa County, Arizona, were attributable to heat by analyzing death certificates. This number of deaths is about 57% more deaths than the 1931 heat-related deaths identified through their physician-certified surveillance system. This gap illustrates how existing heat surveillance approaches may incompletely capture the total heat burden.

POLICY RESPONSES AND PUBLIC HEALTH PRIORITIES

Five editorials are included in this special issue that are policy focused and describe the structural changes needed to combat the threats posed by climate change.

First, Balbus provides a strong defense of the Environmental Protection Agency's 2009 Endangerment Finding for greenhouse gases, which the Trump administration rescinded on February 12, 2026. The Clean Air Act's separation of harm determination from regulatory response has been foundational to its success, saving hundreds of thousands of lives (benefits outweighing costs are 30:1). Balbus frames the rescission as causing psychological trauma for public health professionals and calls for continued scientific documentation, legal support to overturn the rescission, community solidarity, and maintaining hope through evidence-based advocacy.

Second, Ramachandran et al. (p. 769) argue for integrating climate health data into electronic health records to bridge the gap between public health intelligence and clinical care. They describe practical applications such as systems that automatically identify

Continued on page 764...

HISTORY CORNER

61 YEARS AGO

The Clean Air Act and Its Implications

Obviously the Congress in developing the Clean Air Act was aware of the various trends which contribute to a worsening national air pollution problem. . . . But the Clean Air Act was developed in recognition of two other important considerations. First, scientific research has pointed to a strong link between community air pollution and such major diseases of the respiratory system as asthma, bronchitis, emphysema, and probably even the common cold. And second, the cities and states of the nation, upon whom rests the primary responsibility for the regulatory control of air pollution, are not adequately meeting this responsibility. There is consequently a broad need for expansion of control activities, for the attainment of which federal assistance and stimulation can be very helpful and, indeed, are essential.

From *AJPH*, June 1965, p. 901.

high-risk patients during heat advisories coupled with personalized medical advice. This approach transforms passive public health warnings into proactive clinical interventions delivered by trusted care teams.

Third, Sussman (p. 772) portrays the Trump administration's systematic dismantling of climate policy, culminating in the February 2026 repeal of the Environmental Protection Agency's Endangerment Finding. Sussman argues that climate and public health experts must now engage the public directly through media, town halls, and new communication tools to maintain understanding of climate–health connections until policymakers reengage.

Fourth, Sapkota (p. 775) highlights underdiscussed climate-related effects. For example, there is evidence that warming temperatures extend ragweed pollen seasons by up to 27 days, with higher carbon dioxide producing more allergenic pollen, increasing asthma hospitalization risks from both early and late spring onsets. Sapkota calls for bold US climate mitigation action, reinforcing policies such as the Endangerment Finding rather than dismantling them.

Fifth, Jerrett (p. 777) argues that climate-related disasters are now fundamentally "unnatural." Invoking the late Kirk Smith's framework, Jerrett notes that climate change offers three options: mitigate, adapt, or suffer. Current US policy (e.g., Paris Agreement withdrawal, Endangerment Finding rollback, cuts to Federal Emergency Management Agency and Centers for Disease Control and Prevention, elimination of climate research funding), Jerrett asserts, points to increased suffering.

FROM EVIDENCE TO ACTION

Collectively, these contributions demonstrate that climate change operates as a threat multiplier, amplifying existing health inequities through the triple jeopardy of differential exposure, differential susceptibility, and differential adaptive capacity. The editorials and scientific findings suggest several urgent priorities for policy, research, and action. As political attacks on climate science intensify, the public health community must continue to document, analyze, and disseminate evidence on how climate change harms health. The stakes could not be higher: climate change threatens to reverse decades of public health progress and deepen entrenched inequities unless we act decisively to protect the most vulnerable members of our communities. AJPH

CORRESPONDENCE

Correspondence should be sent to Tarik Benmarhnia, PhD, Scripps Institution of Oceanography, University of California, San Diego, 9500 Gilman Dr #0206, La Jolla, CA 92093-0206 (e-mail: tbenmarhnia@ucsd.edu). Reprints can be ordered at https://www.ajph.org by clicking the "Reprints" link.

PUBLICATION INFORMATION

Full Citation: Benmarhnia T, Chartres N. Climate change and health inequities: evidence and action for vulnerable populations. *Am J Public Health*. 2026;116(6):761–764.

Acceptance Date: March 24, 2026.

DOI: https://doi.org/10.2105/AJPH.2026.308561

ORCID iD:
Nicholas Chartres https://orcid.org/0000-0002-9659-6739

CONTRIBUTORS

T. Benmarhnia drafted the initial article. N. Chartres reviewed and edited the article.

ACKNOWLEDGMENTS

We would like to thank Jennifer Schoendorf for the helpful revisions and feedback.

CONFLICTS OF INTEREST

The authors have no conflicts of interest to disclose.

REFERENCES

1. Deivanayagam TA, English S, Hickel J, et al. Envisioning environmental equity: climate change, health, and racial justice. *Lancet*. 2023;402(10395):64–78. https://doi.org/10.1016/S0140-6736(23)00919-4
2. Marlier ME, Connolly R, Ma Y, Jerrett M, Benmarhnia T. Compound climate exposures and public health: a synthesis of research and future directions. *Annu Rev Public Health*. 2025 [Epub ahead of print]. https://doi.org/10.1146/annurev-publhealth-090924-113926
3. Moutet L, Bernard P, Green R, et al. The public health co-benefits of strategies consistent with net-zero emissions: a systematic review. *Lancet Planet Health*. 2025;9(2):e145–e156. https://doi.org/10.1016/S2542-5196(24)00330-9
4. Romanello M, Walawender M, Hsu SC, et al. The 2025 report of the Lancet Countdown on health and climate change: climate change action offers a lifeline. *Lancet*. 2025;406(10521):2804–2857. [Erratum in: *Lancet*. 2025;406(10521):2756. https://doi.org/10.1016/S0140-6736(25)02475-4]. https://doi.org/10.1016/S0140-6736(25)01919-1

Climate Hazards and the Opioid Overdose Epidemic

Joan A. Casey, PhD, Brandon D. L. Marshall, PhD, and Marianthi-Anna Kioumourtzoglou, ScD

ABOUT THE AUTHORS

Joan A. Casey is with the Department of Environmental and Occupational Health Sciences and Epidemiology, School of Public Health, University of Washington, Seattle. Brandon D. L. Marshall is with the Department of Epidemiology, Brown University School of Public Health, Providence, RI. Marianthi-Anna Kioumourtzoglou is with the Department of Epidemiology, Brown University School of Public Health, and the Institute at Brown University for Environment and Society.

See also Climate Change/Natural Disasters, pp. 761–813.

Two worsening crises plague Americans, one fueled by excess carbon dioxide emissions and the other by unregulated synthetic opioids, primarily fentanyl and related analogs. In 2017, the costs of climate disasters in the United States, exclusive of health impacts, totaled $306 billion,[1] and opioid-related mortality and opioid use disorder (OUD) combined exceeded $551 billion.[2]

CLIMATE HAZARDS AND OPIOID-RELATED OVERDOSE

Recent studies reveal increased risk of fatal and nonfatal opioid overdose at higher ambient temperatures[3,4] and after major climactic events, including hurricanes.[5] Evidence suggests that climate change will exacerbate the opioid overdose crisis[6]; hazards such as heatwaves, tropical cyclones, and wildfires can affect the physiology and behavior of people who use drugs (PWUD); cause stress; interrupt the drug supply; increase displacement, social isolation, and housing insecurity; and reduce access to health care, harm reduction services, and other overdose prevention programs (Figure 1). For those with OUD, climate hazards can interrupt access to medications for OUD (MOUD), particularly when opioid treatment programs close or travel to a site becomes unsafe or impossible.[8] PWUD who discontinue MOUD may resume regular use of illicit opioids, doubling or tripling the risk of death immediately following treatment discontinuation.[9] For the 12 million Americans relying on long-term (i.e., > 90-day) prescription opioid therapy, delayed fills could precipitate withdrawal and ultimately increase the risk of unregulated opioid use and overdose.

EXTREME HEAT AND OPIOID-RELATED OVERDOSE

To date, most studies evaluating climate hazards and opioid overdose have focused on extreme heat exposure. Heat exposure can increase the sedative effects of opioids, directly increasing the risk of overdose or reducing the ability of other PWUD to respond to an overdose.[10] Certain combinations of polydrug use (e.g., opioids + amphetamines) can also raise the body's core temperature, increasing odds of overdose,[10] which the urban heat island effect and drug use in buildings or cars without air conditioning can exacerbate.[10] In California, shifting from the 50th to 95th percentile of four-day cumulative average ambient temperature was associated with 8% higher odds of an emergency department visit for opioid overdose.[3] Similarly, in our own research in New York State, we detected nonlinear, increasing associations for opioid-specific hospitalizations for week-long elevated temperatures, and exposure on the day before and day of admission.[11] A 2025 US nationwide study leveraged monthly, county-level, opioid-related mortality rates from 1999 to 2020, and found higher monthly average temperatures associated with additional deaths related to opioids, with heightened effects in counties with higher social vulnerability.[4]

THE ROLE OF OTHER CLIMATE HAZARDS

Different climate hazards may affect opioid overdose differently. Although extreme heat exposure may increase risk of opioid overdose via physiological mechanisms, wildfires and tropical cyclones can worsen mental health; disrupt the unregulated drug market; cause displacement, financial hardship, and deteriorating health; and reduce access to services, thereby indirectly increasing risk of opioid overdose. Wildfire fine particulate matter ($PM_{2.5}$) exposure reduces respiratory function, possibly exacerbating opioid-induced respiratory depression. In British Columbia, same- and next-day ambulance dispatches for cardiac and respiratory arrest increased with wildfire $PM_{2.5}$ levels, with drug overdose a major associated diagnostic code.[12] Although most

AJPH June 2026, Vol. 116, No. 6

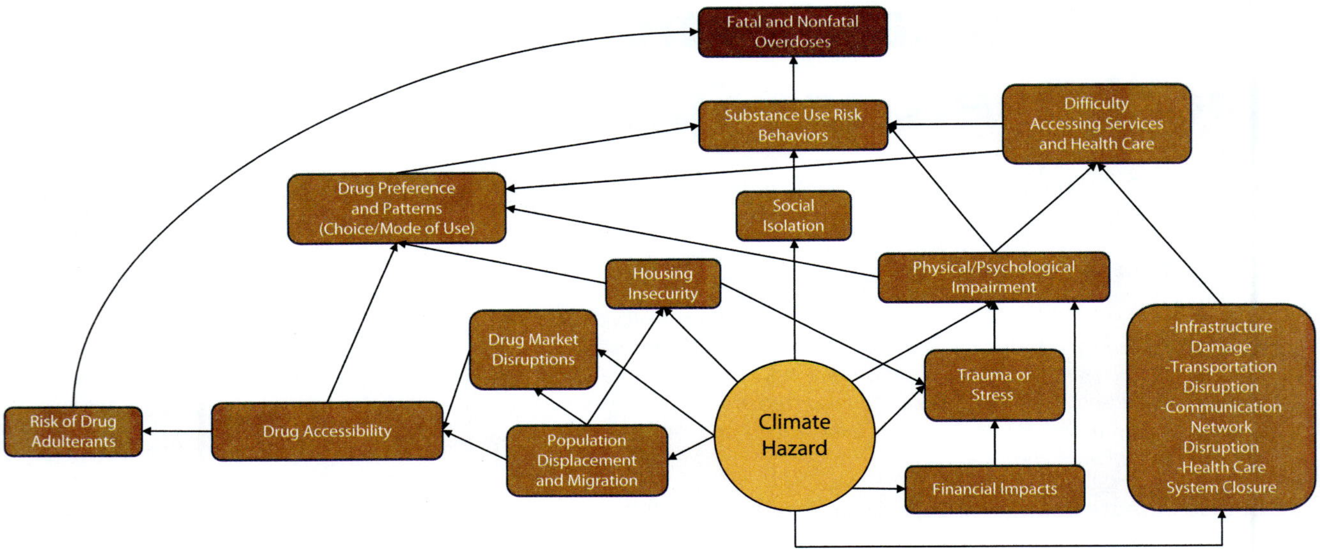

FIGURE 1— Potential Pathways Linking Climate Hazards to Fatal and Nonfatal Opioid Overdose

Note. Not all pathways apply to all climate hazards.
Source. Adapted from Zolopa et al.[7]

studies of tropical cyclone-related risk have focused on small local populations, they have illuminating findings. For instance, 60% of PWUD surveyed in New York City reported experiencing withdrawal in the week following Hurricane Sandy.[13]

RESEARCH NEEDS

Distinct spatiotemporal patterns of the opioid overdose epidemic and climate hazards across the United States necessitate region-specific studies to understand local relationships. Other community characteristics, including factors that influence risk communication, ease of evacuation, and infrastructure and housing resilience, may result in differential impacts (physical, behavioral, and psychological) across climate disaster periods: preparedness, emergency response, recovery, and reconstruction. For example, rural communities may have reduced health care access and longer distances to OUD treatment following a major climatic event (creating barriers to seeking care), whereas tight-knit communities can simultaneously provide support. As climate change intensifies, the prevalence of co-occurring climate hazards (e.g., wildfire + extreme heat) will become more frequent, with potential superadditive impacts on opioid-related overdose that also vary regionally. Analyses elucidating the role of individual and community characteristics may identify important heterogeneities in the relationship between (compound) climate hazard(s) and opioid-related overdose.

To date, population health studies have focused on the impact(s) of short-term (i.e., days to weeks) exposure to climate hazards on changes in drug use behaviors and opioid-related overdose. The few studies examining chronic effects have startling results. Among 66 PWUD in Puerto Rico, the percentage reporting an overdose increased from 10.6% before Hurricane Maria to 24.2% two years after the storm.[5] Fentanyl, damaged infrastructure, and reduced MOUD availability likely explain the increase. Although the risk of opioid-related overdose may peak immediately following climate events, the greatest cumulative effect may occur over the long term, but a gap in research remains.

Beyond assessing the longer-term relationships between climate hazards and overdose, researchers should examine pathways and mechanisms underlying these associations. For people on MOUD—methadone, buprenorphine, and extended-release naltrexone—climate hazards can interrupt treatment, with potential differential impacts by MOUD type. Methadone must be dispensed from a regulated Substance Abuse and Mental Health Service Administration (SAMHSA)-certified opioid treatment program, typically with daily in-person dosing until the onset of COVID-19, when take-home dosing became more common in some states. Conversely, physicians can prescribe or administer extended-release naltrexone (opioid antagonist, monthly injection) in outpatient settings. Given differences in the frequency of (1) interactions between PWUD and treatment providers and (2) treatment administration, it is likely that climate hazards differentially disrupt medication-based therapies. Studies identifying which treatment modality best supports individuals with OUD during and following climate hazards are needed.

OPPORTUNITIES FOR INTERVENTION

Although addressing climate impacts on opioid overdose is a relatively new frontier in public health, some jurisdictions have implemented relevant mitigation policies. For example, some states, including California and Missouri, have implemented regulatory flexibility for medication access and substance use disorder treatment (e.g., telehealth and take-home dosing) in the event of natural disasters.[14] Cities including Phoenix, Arizona and Hartford, Connecticut have begun integrating harm-reduction services into cooling centers, which operate during heat waves. Further evaluation of these policies is needed and should be a research priority. Future efforts should also prioritize locally tailored interventions informed by a clear understanding of the pathways linking climate hazards with opioid overdose. Once key associations are established, characterizing individual- and community-level factors that contribute to observed heterogeneity will help identify locally optimal strategies.

Effective intervention design will require an iterative process involving researchers, local policymakers, and community representatives to strengthen policy relevance and support sustainable, scalable solutions. Such work should be grounded in meaningful, bidirectional engagement, during which research teams listen to locally identified concerns, cogenerate potential solutions, adapt analytic approaches to address them, and share findings that can inform action. Because climate hazards and overdose risks vary across communities, research should include local effect estimation rather than relying solely on state- or national-level analyses, which may mask important local dynamics driven by hazard types or community characteristics. Ultimately, integrating community-based participatory approaches at every step of climate–opioid research will help ensure context-specific, equitable, and feasible interventions.

CONCLUSION

Although research on the intersection of climate hazards and opioid overdoses remains scarce, the escalating threats from both crises underscore the need to prioritize studies that can provide near-term, actionable evidence, including the investigation of causal pathways that are modifiable with public health intervention. AJPH

CORRESPONDENCE

Correspondence should be sent to Joan A. Casey, 3980 15th Ave Northeast, Seattle, WA 98105 (e-mail: jacasey@uw.edu). Reprints can be ordered at https://www.ajph.org by clicking the "Reprints" link.

PUBLICATION INFORMATION

Full Citation: Casey JA, Marshall BDL, Kioumourtzoglou M-A. Climate hazards and the opioid overdose epidemic. *Am J Public Health*. 2026;116(6):765–768.

Acceptance Date: January 21, 2026.

DOI: https://doi.org/10.2105/AJPH.2026.308437

ORCID iD:
Brandon D. L. Marshall https://orcid.org/0000-0002-0134-7052

CONTRIBUTORS

J. A. Casey and M.-A. Kioumourtzoglou generated the original conceptual design. All authors contributed to the original manuscript draft and approved the final version.

ACKNOWLEDGMENTS

This work was supported by the National Institute of Environmental Health Sciences (NIEHS P30 ES007033 [J. A. Casey]) and the National Institute on Aging (NIA P20 AG093975 [M.-A. Kioumourtzoglou]). B. D. L. Marshall is supported in part by a grant from the National Institute of General Medical Sciences (P20 GM125507). Additional funding was provided by the Robert W. Day Endowed Professorship in Public Health (J. A. Casey).

CONFLICTS OF INTEREST

The authors have no conflicts of interest to declare.

REFERENCES

1. Smith A. 2017 US billion-dollar weather and climate disasters: a historic year in context. National Oceanic and Atmospheric Administration. 2018. Available at: https://www.climate.gov/disasters-2017#:~:text=The%20cumulative%20costs%20for%20these,of%20weather%20and%20climate%20disasters. Accessed February 2, 2024.
2. Florence C, Luo F, Rice K. The economic burden of opioid use disorder and fatal opioid overdose in the United States, 2017. *Drug Alcohol Depend.* 2021;218:108350. https://doi.org/10.1016/j.drugalcdep.2020.108350
3. Chang HH, Zhang H, Latimore AD, et al. Associations between short-term ambient temperature exposure and emergency department visits for amphetamine, cocaine, and opioid use in California from 2005 to 2019. *Environ Int.* 2023;181:108233. https://doi.org/10.1016/j.envint.2023.108233
4. Dennett JM, Carrion D, Fiellin DA, Gonsalves GS. Heat exposure and drug overdose mortality in the USA. *Addiction.* 2026;121(2):275–285. https://doi.org/10.1111/add.70191
5. Abadie R, Cano M, Habecker P, Gelpí-Acosta C. Substance use, injection risk behaviors, and fentanyl-related overdose risk among a sample of PWID post-Hurricane Maria. *Harm Reduct J.* 2022;19(1):129. https://doi.org/10.1186/s12954-022-00715-4
6. Vergunst F, Berry HL, Minor K, Chadi N. Climate change and substance-use behaviors: a risk-pathways framework. *Perspect Psychol Sci.* 2023;18(4):936–954. https://doi.org/10.1177/17456916221132739
7. Zolopa C, Hoj S, Bruneau J, et al. A rapid review of the impacts of "Big Events" on risks, harms, and service delivery among people who use drugs: implications for responding to COVID-19. *Int J Drug Policy.* 2021;92:103127. https://doi.org/10.1016/j.drugpo.2021.103127
8. Matusow H, Benoit E, Elliott L, Dunlap E, Rosenblum A. Challenges to opioid treatment programs after Hurricane Sandy: patient and provider perspectives on preparation, impact, and recovery. *Subst Use Misuse.* 2018;53(2):206–219. https://doi.org/10.1080/10826084.2016.1267225

9. Sordo L, Barrio G, Bravo MJ, et al. Mortality risk during and after opioid substitution treatment: systematic review and meta-analysis of cohort studies. *BMJ*. 2017;357:j1550. https://doi.org/10.1136/bmj.j1550
10. Ryus C, Bernstein SL. A new syndemic: complications of opioid use disorder during a heat wave. *J Health Care Poor Underserved*. 2022;33(3):1671–1677. https://doi.org/10.1353/hpu.2022.0092
11. Parks RM, Rowland ST, Do V, et al. The association between temperature and alcohol- and substance-related disorder hospital visits in New York State. *Commun Med (Lond)*. 2023;3(1):118. https://doi.org/10.1038/s43856-023-00346-1
12. Yao J, Brauer M, Wei J, McGrail KM, Johnston FH, Henderson SB. Sub-daily exposure to fine particulate matter and ambulance dispatches during wildfire seasons: a case-crossover study in British Columbia, Canada. *Environ Health Perspect*. 2020;128(6):67006.
13. Pouget ER, Sandoval M, Nikolopoulos GK, Friedman SR. Immediate impact of Hurricane Sandy on people who inject drugs in New York City. *Subst Use Misuse*. 2015;50(7):878–884. https://doi.org/10.3109/10826084.2015.978675
14. Suen L, Roberts K, Luba R. Climate disasters create life-threatening disruptions for people on methadone. 2025. Available at: https://www.statnews.com/2025/07/23/methadone-clinics-otp-climate-disaster-disrupted-treatment-texas-floods-hurricane-helene. Accessed January 8, 2026.

From Silos to Systems: Leveraging Technology to Bring Climate Health Insights to the Bedside and Back

Anu Ramachandran, MD, MPH, Arianne Teherani, PhD, and Sheri D. Weiser, MD, MPH

ABOUT THE AUTHORS

Anu Ramachandran is with the Division of Occupational, Environmental, and Climate Medicine and the Department of Emergency Medicine, University of California, San Francisco. Arianne Teherani and Sheri D. Weiser are with the Department of Medicine, University of California, San Francisco.

See also Climate Change/Natural Disasters, pp. 761–813.

The accelerating impacts of climate change pose an urgent threat to human health.[1] Rising temperatures, escalating extreme weather events, and worsening air quality are driving morbidity and mortality ranging from cardiovascular and respiratory illness to mental health emergencies, vector-borne diseases and adverse pregnancy outcomes, impacts inequitably borne by disadvantaged populations.[1] Hospitals and clinicians are at the frontlines of this change, adapting treatment strategies to meet escalating needs. Yet a critical gap exists between climate disaster resources generated by public health agencies and the providers who directly care for those at risk. Tools such as exposure modeling and resource mapping remain inaccessible at the point of care, where treatment decisions are made.[2] Concurrently, insights from providers treating climate-related diseases or testing risk-mitigation interventions are rarely available to inform public health responses.

These silos create a profound disconnect. Public health agencies invest substantial resources creating high-quality climate health information that fails to reach vulnerable patients when they need it most, because we have not invested in the infrastructure to deliver these resources to clinicians effectively, or to relay clinical data back to public health agencies.[2,3] With rapid technological innovation transforming health care delivery—from electronic health records (EHRs) to artificial intelligence–supported clinical decision support systems—we have an unprecedented opportunity to bring critical public health information to and from the bedside and protect health during climate emergencies. We argue that bidirectional data infrastructure linking public health climate intelligence with EHRs is essential to equitable, scalable, and evidence-generating care.

PHYSICIANS ARE TRUSTED BUT UNDERTRAINED AND UNDERRESOURCED

Clinicians are among the most trusted sources of climate health information.[4] Early evidence suggests this counseling is both desired by patients and effective at influencing health-protective behaviors, with families across the political spectrum reporting increased knowledge and behavior change following climate health discussions with their physicians.[5,6]

Despite this potential, clinicians face a profound knowledge gap, undermining their ability to fulfill this role. Although 93% of recently surveyed health professionals considered climate change highly relevant, only 12% felt well-informed in counseling patients.[7] Yet escalating and competing demands on time make it challenging to add climate counseling to already-packed visits without structural support.

BIDIRECTIONAL TECHNOLOGY INFRASTRUCTURE

Technology can bridge the gap between public health insights and bedside care.[5,8] Although current EHRs do not integrate environmental data, the infrastructure exists to do so, and demand is strong: 71% of surveyed clinician informatics specialists wanted climate health information included in EHRs.[9] The technological pathway builds on existing EHR capabilities and established interoperability standards.[8] The standards that enable clinical data exchange can facilitate bidirectional climate–health information: environmental exposure data flowing into clinical workflows, and de-identified outcomes flowing back to public health agencies to strengthen population-level interventions.

This approach transforms the clinician's role from isolated expert to conduit for sophisticated climate health intelligence, while contributing to the

AJPH June 2026, Vol. 116, No. 6

evidence base informing public health responses. Rather than physicians remembering heat-sensitive medications or vulnerability drivers, the EHR flags risks automatically and suggests concrete steps, complementing programs to build provider awareness and education. The goal is to transform passive public health warnings into proactive, personalized interventions delivered at the point of care.

INTEGRATED CLINICAL OUTREACH DURING CLIMATE EMERGENCIES

Linkage of real-time exposure information with clinical data enables scalable, automated outreach during climate emergencies. When a heat advisory is issued or air quality deteriorates, decision-support systems can automatically identify high-risk patients based on medical comorbidities, prescriptions, or key social vulnerabilities. These systems alert and educate providers while triggering interventions: reminding patients to refill inhalers, providing directions to local cooling centers, or delivering resources for shelter or urgent mental health support.

This approach reinforces existing public health infrastructure, transforming population-level warnings into clinically tailored, patient-specific interventions delivered by trusted care teams. Efforts to date include heat-triggered clinic outreach to pregnant patients,[10] climate action plans for community clinics,[11] and integrating air quality sensing into health records for emphysema patients,[12] among others. Building on this foundation, ongoing work at the University of California, San Francisco, is developing scalable EHR-integrated tools to combine high-risk patient registries with real-time temperature and air quality data to develop customized alerts and pilot outreach strategies. Initial pilots include clinically tailored recommendations (such as a patient's personalized asthma action plan or counseling on dehydration risk for those on diuretics) paired with address-based local public health resources. Once the basic infrastructure is developed, tools can be adapted to different clinical contexts or interventions, such as triggering home health visits for highly vulnerable patients or integrating services from local community-based organizations supporting climate resiliency.

FROM THE BEDSIDE BACK TO PUBLIC HEALTH

Returning de-identified clinical data to public health agencies is equally critical. EHRs contain a wealth of information about climate-related health impacts that, when aggregated, could strengthen public health surveillance, resource allocation, intervention evaluation, and policy advocacy.

EHR-based surveillance provides rapidly updated data on diverse health outcomes at finer geographic levels than traditional systems. The Electronic Medical Record Support for Public Health platform demonstrates this potential: the system extracts raw data from EHRs, identifies conditions of public health interest, and communicates results to state health departments, without changing clinical workflows. These data augment existing surveillance and allow allocation of limited resources to highest-impact areas. Linkage of these data also enables more rigorous evaluation and refinement of public health strategies. Finally, robust data on the clinical impacts observed during these events, and the granular risk stratification possible with EHRs, can inform policy and advocacy to improve investments in public health climate resiliency.

CALL TO ACTION

Building climate resilience into the infrastructure of health care delivery as a foundational capability will require collaboration between public health agencies, health systems, informatics leaders, and policymakers.

Public health agencies must lead in developing the data infrastructure that makes bidirectional exchange possible. This includes standardized agreements that make critical information, such as heat advisories, vulnerability maps, and community resources, accessible to clinical systems in real time, along with the infrastructure to receive and integrate clinical data. The Centers for Disease Control and Prevention's National Environmental Public Health Tracking Program and Building Resilience Against Climate Effects (BRACE) framework provide foundations, but these efforts must be resourced and prioritized at multiple levels.

Health systems must invest in infrastructure that integrates climate data into clinical decision tools and outreach strategies. Major EHR vendors should prioritize environmental data integration into core functionality. Health systems must commit to sharing appropriately de-identified data back to public health partners to enable continuous improvement.

Policymakers can accelerate adoption through incentives such as quality measures or reimbursement structures that recognize climate-informed care. Of particular importance in the current federal landscape is empowering state and local governments to support public health agencies and mandate data-sharing agreements that enable bidirectional exchange.

Finally, researchers must build the evidence base for interventions translating climate warnings into population health benefits. Frameworks such as the Consolidated Framework for Implementation Research can guide efforts to identify barriers and facilitate the adoption of climate-informed practices.

CONCLUSION

Climate change is already driving increased mortality worldwide. The health sector cannot afford to wait. By building bidirectional data infrastructure that connects public health tools with clinical insights, we can transform fragmented responses into coordinated, proactive, and equitable protection, saving lives by ensuring that climate health information reaches the people who need it, through the providers they trust, at the moment it matters most. AJPH

CORRESPONDENCE

Correspondence should be sent to Anu Ramachandran, MD, MPH, 505 Parnassus Ave, San Francisco, CA 94143 (e-mail: anu.ramachandran@ucsf.edu). Reprints can be ordered at https://www.ajph.org by clicking the "Reprints" link.

PUBLICATION INFORMATION

Full Citation: Ramachandran A, Teherani A, Weiser SD. From silos to systems: leveraging technology to bring climate health insights to the bedside and back. *Am J Public Health.* 2026;116(6):769–771.

Acceptance Date: March 18, 2026

DOI: https://doi.org/10.2105/AJPH.2026.308545

ORCID iDs:

Anu Ramachandran https://orcid.org/0009-0002-6413-9493

Arianne Teherani https://orcid.org/0000-0003-2936-9832

CONTRIBUTORS

A. Ramachandran was responsible for manuscript drafting. A. Teherani and S. D. Weiser critically revised the manuscript. All authors contributed to the conceptualization of this work and approved the final version for publication.

CONFLICTS OF INTEREST

The authors declare no conflicts of interest.

REFERENCES

1. Romanello M, McGushin A, Di Napoli C, et al. The 2021 report of the Lancet Countdown on health and climate change: code red for a healthy future. *Lancet.* 2021;398(10311):1619–1662. https://doi.org/10.1016/S0140-6736(21)01787-6
2. Walker DM, Yeager VA, Lawrence J, McAlearney AS. Identifying opportunities to strengthen the public health informatics infrastructure: exploring hospitals' challenges with data exchange. *Milbank Q.* 2021;99(2):393–425. https://doi.org/10.1111/1468-0009.12511
3. Dzau VJ, McClellan MB, McGinnis JM, et al. Vital directions for health and health care: priorities from a National Academy of Medicine initiative. *JAMA.* 2017;317(14):1461–1470. https://doi.org/10.1001/jama.2017.1964
4. Wellbery CE, Lewandowski A, Holder C. Climate change and the local environment: communicating with your patients about health impacts. *Am Fam Physician.* 2021;104(5):526–530. Available at: https://www.aafp.org/pubs/afp/issues/2021/1100/p526.html. Accessed April 7, 2026.
5. McLellan RK, Berenji M, Egbuji A, et al. Harnessing occupational and environmental medicine expertise to transform medical care: a catalyst for mitigating the human health impacts of climate change. *J Occup Environ Med.* 2025;67(10):e743–e758. https://doi.org/10.1097/JOM.0000000000003523
6. Uppalapati SSS, Ansah POO, Campbell E, et al. A global review of research on effective advocacy and communication strategies at the intersection of climate change and health. George Mason University. 2023. Available at: https://climatecommunication.gmu.edu/wp-content/uploads/2023/11/Climate-and-Health-Literature-Review-Final.pdf. Accessed March 9, 2026.
7. Albrecht L, Reismann L, Leitzmann M, et al. Climate-specific health literacy in health professionals: an exploratory study. *Front Med (Lausanne).* 2023;10:1236319. https://doi.org/10.3389/fmed.2023.1236319
8. Akras Z, Dresser C, Ashworth H. Integration of environmental data into electronic health records for clinical and public health decision making: a viewpoint on expanding development in the United States. *J Med Internet Res.* 2025;27:e76396. https://doi.org/10.2196/76396
9. Sarabu C, Deonarine A, Leitner S, Fayanju O, Fisun M, Nadeau K. Climate change and health informatics: pilot survey of perspectives across the field. *J Am Med Inform Assoc.* 2022;29(12):2117–2123. https://doi.org/10.1093/jamia/ocac199
10. National Association of Community Health Centers. Heat related messaging highlight—La Clinica. 2024 Available at: https://www.nachc.org/about-nachc/our-work/air-water-and-chemical-exposures/heat-and-health-basics/heat-related-messaging-highlight-la-clinica. Accessed March 8, 2026.
11. Nayak A. Amid extreme heat, this program tackles climate change with heat action clinics. *JAMA.* 2025;334(9):753–754. https://doi.org/10.1001/jama.2025.11906
12. Kuhn BT, Gupta R. Improving wildfire readiness among patients with chronic obstructive pulmonary disease and asthma: applying a population health approach to climate change. *Chronic Obstr Pulm Dis.* 2024;11(4):427–435. https://doi.org/10.15326/jcopdf.2024.0509

Returning Public Health to the National Conversation on Climate Change

Robert Sussman, JD

ABOUT THE AUTHOR

Robert Sussman is a lawyer and former Environmental Protection Agency official with the law and policy firm Sussman & Associates, Washington, DC.

See also Climate Change/Natural Disasters, pp. 761–813.

AJPH June 2026, Vol. 116, No. 6

Reversing decades of climate policy, our national leaders have decided that climate change is a nonproblem and (to quote President Trump) a "hoax" and a "scam." At the direction of the president and his top officials, the United States has disengaged from global action to address planetary warming. This pullback has occurred across all government programs. In a little over a year, the United States has withdrawn from the foundational international agreements that call for cooperative efforts to reduce emissions of heat-trapping gases; eliminated research on the causes and consequences of global warming; abandoned joint efforts by the world's leading experts to advance climate science; and discouraged wind, solar, electric vehicles, and other nonemitting technologies while promoting fossil fuels that not only accelerate climate change but have well-recognized harmful effects on our health.[1]

ABANDONING THE ENDANGERMENT FINDING

The common denominator of these efforts has been indifference to science and public health. There is a mass of scientific evidence demonstrating the myriad ways a warming planet is a threat to our health and well-being, but this evidence has been derided and ignored by those who now set national policy.

The latest domino to fall was the February 12, 2026, repeal by the Environmental Protection Agency (EPA) of its landmark 2009 Endangerment Finding.[2] For the past 16 years, this decision has been the cornerstone of US actions under the Clean Air Act to reduce emissions of greenhouse gases, whose buildup in the atmosphere is causing rising global temperatures. Because of these and other actions, US greenhouse gas emissions fell by 17% between 2005 and 2022.[3]

SCIENTIFIC BASIS OF THE ENDANGERMENT FINDING

The Endangerment Finding responded to the 2007 Supreme Court decision in *Massachusetts v EPA* (549 US 497; 2007), a case seeking to enforce the EPA's obligation to limit greenhouse gas emissions from motor vehicles because of their contribution to climate change.[4] The Supreme Court sided with the challengers, determining that these gases were "pollutants" no different from particulate matter and ozone, whose emissions had long been controlled under the Clean Air Act because of their known adverse effects on health. Recognizing that "the harms associated with climate change are serious and well recognized" and include "increases in the spread of disease," the court held that the EPA was required by the act to reduce vehicle greenhouse gas emissions if they "cause, or contribute to, air pollution which may reasonably be anticipated to endanger public health or welfare."[4] To make this determination, the court called on the EPA to make a science-based judgment on whether "sufficient information demonstrates" that the contribution of vehicle emissions to climate change is harming public health and welfare.[4]

The EPA took this charge seriously by conducting a comprehensive review of the scientific literature and assigning principal weight to the findings of three prestigious scientific bodies: the US Global Climate Research Program, the Intergovernmental Panel on Climate Change, and the National Research Council. Like these other bodies, the EPA's scientific review concluded, "The evidence provides compelling support for finding that greenhouse gas air pollution endangers the public welfare of both current and future generations"[5(p66498)] and the "risk and the severity of adverse impacts on public welfare are expected to increase over time."[5(p66499)]

Elaborating, the EPA cited several harmful consequences of climate change. For example, it found that "increases in ambient ozone are expected to occur over broad areas of the country, and [will] increase serious adverse health effects in large population areas."[5(p66497)] It also found that "increases in average temperatures, which increase the likelihood of heat waves" will result in greater "mortality and morbidity."[5(p66497)] And it pointed to "numerous and far-ranging risks to food production and agriculture, forestry, water resources, sea level rise and coastal areas [and] energy infrastructure"[5(p66498)] and emphasized that "the evidence concerning how human-induced climate change may alter extreme weather events also clearly supports a finding of endangerment, given the serious adverse impacts that can result from such events."[5(p66497)]

TRUMP'S FAILED ATTACK ON THE SCIENCE

Since 2009, the frequency and severity of droughts, extreme weather events, sea-level rise, ice pack melting, flooding, destructive wildfires, and heat-induced mortality have increased, validating the Endangerment Finding's predictions.[6] But the administration's starting point for repealing the finding was that these alarming trends were not real and that the EPA's 2009 scientific review was based on flawed and incomplete evidence. Anticipating that it would be able to demolish the scientific case for climate change, the EPA administrator promised to drive "a dagger straight into the heart of the climate change religion"[(https://bit.ly/3NTNLXR)] and eliminate its "holy grail."[7] But this turned out to be an empty promise. When push came to shove, the administration was unable to mount a credible critique of mainstream climate science and was forced to abort the effort after critics charged that it lacked objectivity, balance, and transparency.

The scientific community might well have supported an unbiased, nonpolitical process to reexamine the scientific evidence for global warming. But taking no chances, the administration instead commissioned a report from five climate deniers who were selected in secret and deliberated behind closed doors.[8] They failed to consult the hundreds of career climate experts at the National Oceanic and Atmospheric Administration, the National Aeronautics and Space Administration, and the EPA and bypassed the rigorous peer review process for scientific assessments supporting major policy decisions. Irate about the report's one-sided findings, 85 well-known climate scientists issued a statement rejecting its conclusions as "misleading or fundamentally incorrect."[9]

The National Academy of Sciences, Engineering, and Medicine then weighed in with its own independent, self-funded review of the climate science published since 2009 and submitted it to the EPA. The academy concluded that evidence of harm to human health and welfare from climate change "is beyond scientific dispute" and that "much of the understanding of climate change that was uncertain or tentative in 2009 has now been resolved" and new threats have been identified.[10]

FALLING BACK ON LEGALISMS

Backed into a corner, the administration removed any discussion of climate science and public health from its final rationale for repealing the Endangerment Finding.[2] Instead, it relied entirely on claimed errors in the *Massachusetts v EPA* decision and the EPA's previous interpretation of its legal authority. This shift from attacking the science to ignoring it put the administration in the untenable position of tacitly admitting that it could not disprove climate change's effects on public health and welfare but that the science ultimately did not matter because the Clean Air Act never authorized the Endangerment Finding to begin with.

Lawyers are now gearing up to debate the legal merits of this position, and ultimately the Supreme Court may need to once again clarify the law. But as the court cases proceed, the public conversation about climate science and its implications for public health and welfare has been left hanging. Most likely, the administration will continue to claim that climate concerns have no basis in reality and are the invention of overzealous advocates. But because the administration's attack on the science has not been put to a decisive test in a credible scientific forum, the public may be confused and uncertain about what to believe.

ROLE OF SCIENCE AND PUBLIC HEALTH IN PUBLIC ENGAGEMENT

At this moment of uncertainty, climate and public health experts must play a bigger role in keeping the public engaged and ensuring that climate-driven impacts on public health and welfare are understood not as isolated events but as the result of global climate trends that societies must address. Our leading experts have fought hard to defend climate science in academic journals and formal submissions to government bodies but have been less successful in translating the science into understandable messages that wider audiences can grasp and relate to daily life. This must change. Scientists are often uncomfortable in the role of communicators and advocates but, at a time when many public officials have been silenced, they may be the only remaining source of trustworthy and objective information and advice that can sway the public. If they do not use their knowledge of the science to educate the citizenry about climate change, there will be no respected voice to counter the incendiary and misleading rhetoric of the administration. The stakes are too high for scientists to remain on the sidelines and let others control the debate.

Maintaining a vibrant public discussion of climate change will require climate scientists to join forces with public health experts to reach new audiences. This entails publicizing new scientific findings and using new communication tools to explain their significance. Scientists must seek out the media to keep climate issues on the front burner and use town hall meetings, op-eds, teach-ins, and other outlets to present the science to communities and demonstrate its relevance to their lives.

Despite the discouraging setbacks of the Trump administration, it is only a matter of time before policymakers reengage on climate and again look for solutions. Scientists and public health experts must now lay the foundation to meet this challenge when it comes. AJPH

CORRESPONDENCE

Correspondence should be sent to Robert Sussman, Sussman & Associates, 3101 Garfield St NW, Washington, DC 20008 (e-mail: bobsussman1@comcast.net). Reprints can be ordered at https://www.ajph.org by clicking the "Reprints" link.

PUBLICATION INFORMATION

Full Citation: Sussman R. Returning public health to the national conversation on climate change. *Am J Public Health*. 2026;116(6):772–774.

Acceptance Date: March 20, 2026.

DOI: https://doi.org/10.2105/AJPH.2026.308551

CONFLICTS OF INTEREST

The author has no conflicts of interest to report.

REFERENCES

1. Environmental Law Institute. The anti-climate fanaticism of the second Trump term. 2024. Available at: https://www.eli.org/vibrant-environment-blog/anti-climate-fanaticism-second-trump-term. Accessed March 29, 2026.
2. US Environmental Protection Agency. Rescission of the greenhouse gas endangerment finding and motor vehicle greenhouse gas emission standards under the Clean Air Act. *Fed Regist.* 2026;91(32):7686–7796.
3. US Environmental Protection Agency. Inventory of US greenhouse gas emissions and sinks: 1990–2022. March 6, 2026. Available at: https://www.epa.gov/ghgemissions/inventory-us-greenhouse-gas-emissions-and-sinks-1990-2022. Accessed March 29, 2026.
4. Justia. *Massachusetts v EPA*, 549 U.S. 497 (2007). 2007. Available at: https://supreme.justia.com/cases/federal/us/549/497. Accessed March 29, 2026.
5. US Environmental Protection Agency. 40 CFR Chapter I. Endangerment and cause or contribute findings for greenhouse gases under Section 202(A) of the Clean Air Act. *Fed Regist.* 2009; 74(239):66496–66546.
6. Danielle M. Warming atmosphere fueling heavier US rainfall and rising flood risk, AccuWeather analysis shows. September 19, 2025. Available at: https://www.accuweather.com/en/weather-news/warming-atmosphere-fueling-heavier-u-s-rainfall-and-rising-flood-risk-accuweather-analysis-shows/1814984. Accessed March 29, 2026.
7. Chemnick J. Breaking down Zeldin's rollbacks. March 13, 2025. Available at: https://www.eenews.net/articles/breaking-down-zeldins-rollbacks. Accessed March 25, 2026.
8. US Department of Energy. A critical review of impacts of greenhouse gas emissions on the US climate. 2025. Available at: https://www.energy.gov/sites/default/files/2025-07/DOE_Critical_Review_of_Impacts_of_greenhousegas_Emissions_on_the_US_Climate_July_2025.pdf. Accessed March 29, 2026.
9. Dessler A, Kopp RE. Climate experts' review of the DOE climate working group report. September 29, 2025. Available at: https://doi.org/10.22541/essoar.175745244.41950365/v2. Accessed March 29, 2026.
10. National Academies of Sciences, Engineering, and Medicine. National academies publish new report reviewing evidence for greenhouse gas emissions and US climate, health, and welfare. September 17, 2025. Available at: https://www.nationalacademies.org/news/national-academies-publish-new-report-reviewing-evidence-for-greenhouse-gas-emissions-and-u-s-climate-health-and-welfare. Accessed March 29, 2026.

Understudied Climate Change Attributes and Health Threats

Amir Sapkota, PhD

ABOUT THE AUTHOR

Amir Sapkota is with the Department of Epidemiology and Biostatistics, University of Maryland School of Public Health, College Park.

See also Climate Change/Natural Disasters, pp. 761–813.

The Ellicott City–Baltimore/Washington International Airport area in my home state of Maryland experienced a "once in a thousand-year rainfall event" (with < 0.1% chance of happening in any given year) in August 2014,[1] July 2016, and yet again in May 2018.[2] Such extreme weather events, including heat waves, droughts, and wildfires, are becoming more common, more intense, and longer lasting.[3] Climate scientists now agree that this increasing frequency of extreme weather events is tied to anthropogenic climate change.[3]

A large body of literature has documented both the direct and indirect impacts of extreme weather events on public health. Less discussed are the more subtle attributes of climate change that can negatively affect health. One such example is the intricate relationship between warming temperature, plant phenology, and burden of allergic diseases. Just as human physiology is closely regulated by circadian rhythm with light as its environmental cue, plant phenology (timing of seed germination, onset of spring, flowering, fall senescence) is influenced by the ambient temperature. Warming temperature has been linked to lengthening of the fall ragweed pollen season by as much as 27 days,[4] in some cases extending into the winter. Unusually warm (cold) wintertime temperatures can lead to earlier (late) onset of spring across North America. Early onset of spring can increase the length of tree pollen season in the spring, whereas late onset can increase the effective pollen concentration in the environment because of the multiple species of trees blooming together. Previous studies have shown that both early and late onset of spring can increase the risk of asthma hospitalization.[5] In addition, plants like ragweed are known to produce higher concentrations of pollen and more allergenic pollen under higher CO_2 concentrations and warmer temperatures, further amplifying the risk of allergic disease.

Likewise, ongoing climate change is disrupting monsoon dynamics (e.g., timing of monsoon onset, withdrawal, intensity, and season length), a key driver of agricultural productivity in large swaths of the world. Rice farmers in Asia closely synchronize their rice planting to coincide with the arrival of seasonal monsoon rain, which is critical for seed germination and early crop growth. For this reason, both early and late monsoon arrival can significantly disrupt the planting schedules, resulting in crop failure. As such, changes in the timing of monsoon onset not only affect farmers financially but also increase the risk of malnutrition, compromising health and well-being.[6] Previous studies have shown that higher concentrations of CO_2 can reduce the nutritional content, such as protein, iron, and zinc, in staple crops.[7] Given that the vast majority of the global population receives its largest share of nutrients from plant-based diets (protein: 63%; iron: 81%; zinc: 68%), ongoing climate change has the potential to increase the severity of nutritional deficiencies,[7] with disproportionate impacts among pregnant women and young children.

Although the impacts of extreme heat exposures on public health have been studied extensively, less discussed are its detrimental impacts among highly vulnerable populations, such as migrant workers from low- and middle-income countries. A large number of migrant workers from South Asian countries, including Nepal, Bangladesh, India, and Sri Lanka, travel to Persian Gulf nations in search of economic opportunities. Many of them end up working outdoors in extreme desert heat with limited access to shade, rest, and hydration.[8] Emerging evidence suggests that such occupational exposures to extreme heat combined with chronic dehydration may lead to the development of chronic kidney disease, which can progress to end-stage kidney disease, requiring dialysis.[9] In fact, a recent study from Nepal found that 31% of dialysis patients at a treatment center were returnee migrant workers from Gulf countries.[10] A separate study reported that more than 50% of returnee migrant workers who received kidney transplants had worked outdoors in extreme desert heat exceeding 40°C to 50°C.[8] The *Kafala* system practiced in

AJPH June 2026, Vol. 116, No. 6

many Gulf countries restricts workers from switching jobs without explicit approval from their employer, leaving many migrant workers helpless. Once diagnosed with kidney failure, the workers, often in their early 30s, are sent home, where they must rely on long-term dialysis.[8]

Whether it is a rural farming family facing malnutrition or migrant workers losing kidney function, poor and marginalized communities, who have contributed the least to the greenhouse gas emissions responsible for climate change, are often the ones facing the disproportionate burden of health threats from climate change. The threat faced by affected individuals can exact significant financial and mental health tolls among family members as well. For example, dialysis centers in Nepal are largely concentrated in major cities, far from the rural villages where many migrant workers' families live. As a result, families are often forced to rent small rooms in the city—an expense they can scarcely afford—so that their loved ones can access life-saving dialysis treatment two to three times a week.

Although some of the examples used to highlight the subtle and less discussed health threats of climate change are from across the globe, communities across the United States are facing analogous threats. Ultimately, a healthier America and a prosperous America are two sides of the same coin that go hand in hand. American leaders throughout history have risen to the occasion to build both, implementing policies that have not only turned burning rivers[11] to recreational oases but also reduced putrid air quality that was killing Americans en masse[12] to among the best in the world. At present, climate change represents humanity's grand challenge, requiring an unwavering commitment to address it so we can protect the health and well-being of all Americans. The ongoing work on carbon capture technology is praiseworthy; it would be a mistake, however, and unfair to pin all of humanity's hope on yet unproven technologies to solve this grand challenge. Although public health communities across the country are working to strengthen adaptation strategies to reduce extreme weather–related morbidity and mortality, the United States needs its leaders to take bold action on climate mitigation. This includes reinforcing and improving existing policies such as the Environmental Protection Agency's 2009 Endangerment Finding—which, although imperfect, has demonstrated effectiveness in reducing greenhouse gas emissions—rather than dismantling them. AJPH

CORRESPONDENCE

Correspondence should be sent to Amir Sapkota, PhD, Department of Epidemiology and Biostatistics, University of Maryland School of Public Health, Room 1340G Atlantic Bldg, College Park, MD 20742 (e-mail: amirsap@umd.edu). Reprints can be ordered at https://www.ajph.org by clicking the "Reprints" link.

PUBLICATION INFORMATION

Full Citation: Sapkota A. Understudied climate change attributes and health threats. *Am J Public Health*. 2026;116(6):775–776.

Acceptance Date: March 18, 2026

DOI: https://doi.org/10.2105/AJPH.2026.308547

ORCID iD:

Amir Sapkota https://orcid.org/0000-0001-5978-2543

CONFLICTS OF INTEREST

The author has no conflicts of interest to declare.

REFERENCES

1. Samenow J. Weather Service: BWI witnessed "between a 500 year and 1,000 year rainfall." *Washington Post*. August 14, 2014. Available at: https://www.washingtonpost.com/news/capital-weather-gang/wp/2014/08/14/weather-service-bwi-witnessed-between-a-500-year-and-1000-year-rainfall. Accessed March 5, 2026.
2. di Liberto T. Torrential rains bring epic flash floods in Maryland in late May 2018. Climate.gov. 2018. Available at: https://www.climate.gov/news-features/event-tracker/torrential-rains-bring-epic-flash-floods-maryland-late-may-2018. Accessed March 5, 2026.
3. *Fifth National Climate Assessment*. Washington, DC: US Global Change Research Program; 2023.
4. Ziska L, Knowlton K, Rogers C, et al. Recent warming by latitude associated with increased length of ragweed pollen season in central North America. *Proc Natl Acad Sci U S A*. 2011;108(10):4248–4251. https://doi.org/10.1073/pnas.1014107108
5. Sapkota A, Dong Y, Li L, et al. association between changes in timing of spring onset and asthma hospitalization in Maryland. *JAMA Netw Open*. 2020;3(7):e207551. https://doi.org/10.1001/jamanetworkopen.2020.7551
6. Thiede BC, Gray C. Climate exposures and child undernutrition: evidence from Indonesia. *Soc Sci Med*. 2020;265:113298. https://doi.org/10.1016/j.socscimed.2020.113298
7. Ziska LH. Rising carbon dioxide and global nutrition: evidence and action needed. *Plants (Basel)*. 2022;11(7):1000. https://doi.org/10.3390/plants11071000
8. Shrestha PC, Bogati C, Shrestha P, Tuladhar SR, Shrestha KK. Kidney transplants in Nepali migrant workers: health and employment insights. *Ann Med Surg (Lond)*. 2025;87(10):6346–6351. https://doi.org/10.1097/MS9.0000000000003828
9. Nerbass FB, Pecoits-Filho R, Clark WF, Sontrop JM, McIntyre CW, Moist L. Occupational heat stress and kidney health: from farms to factories. *Kidney Int Rep*. 2017;2(6):998–1008. https://doi.org/10.1016/j.ekir.2017.08.012
10. Sharma SK, Upadhyaya MK. Migrant work and kidney health in Nepal: prevention is better than cure. *Kidney360*. 2024;5(10):1563–1565. https://doi.org/10.34067/KID.0000000000000550
11. Adler JH. Fables of the Cuyahoga: reconstructing a history of environmental protection. *Fordham Environ Law J*. 2002. Available at: https://scholarlycommons.law.case.edu/faculty_publications/191. Accessed March 5, 2026.
12. Townsend JG. Investigation of the smog incident in Donora, Pa., and vicinity. *Am J Public Health Nations Health*. 1950;40(2):183–189. https://doi.org/10.2105/ajph.40.2.183

Public Health Endangerment From Climate Change and Unnatural Disasters in the Anthropocene

Michael Jerrett, PhD

ABOUT THE AUTHOR

The author is with the Center for Healthy Climate Solutions the Department of Environmental Health Sciences, Fielding School of Public Health, University of California, Los Angeles.

See also Climate Change/Natural Disasters, pp. 761–813.

In March 2024, the International Commission on Stratigraphy rejected a proposal to recognize the Anthropocene as an official geological epoch, a contested, controversial decision.[1] Nevertheless, the concept remains a powerful heuristic for understanding the impact of the pervasive and now dominant influence of human activities on planet Earth. Nowhere is this truer than with the human influence on global climate, with the myriad of regional effects manifest in extreme weather and related disasters. From a public health perspective, as evidenced by the articles in this special issue, many of the projected health effects of climate change are already upon us. Disasters such as extreme weather events (both powerful storms and extreme heat) and wildfires (e.g., the massive conflagrations in Los Angeles in 2025, with toxic pollutants affecting millions during the fires and for many months afterward[2,3]) present huge threats to public health in the United States and around the world. As with so many climate-related disasters, these events all have a human imprimatur.

In the South Coast region, for example, which includes Los Angeles, 98% of wildfire ignitions are now of human origin.[4] Such statistics remind us of the "unnatural" or anthropogenic origin of these classified "natural disasters." Although extreme heat, wildfires, and severe storms have occurred for millennia, human-induced climate change and related environmental mismanagement contribute to the increased size, frequency, and severity of these disasters. Thus, in the era of the Anthropocene, with massive and accelerating changes in the climate, many disasters previously thought of as natural have become decidedly unnatural. It is virtually unequivocal that human activities, particularly fossil fuel combustion, principally drive climate change and many of the ensuing health risks.[5]

Climate change now interacts with other drivers, such as poorly managed development at the wildland–urban interface; part of this stems from people seeking affordable housing because they have been outpriced in urban areas.[6] The synergisms among the housing affordability crisis, climate change, and wildfire risk fall under a broader conceptualization of a "syndemic," meaning that the changing climate interacts with and multiplies the risks of many other major problems of our time with the result being heightened disease incidence.[7]

What will the acceleration of unnatural disasters mean for public health? When I taught a graduate course on climate change and public health at the University of California, Berkeley, with the now dearly departed Kirk Smith, he would always explain to the students that climate change presented us with three options: mitigate emissions to lessen the damage, adapt and build community resilience, or suffer. The withdrawal of the United States from the 2015 Paris Agreement on climate change and the World Health Organization, the recent rollback of the endangerment finding that empowered the US Environmental Protection Agency to regulate greenhouse gas emissions (along with the promise not to enforce the major regulations it empowered), huge spending cuts on federal programs designed to build community resilience with adaptive measures, the unprecedented decline in support for research on climate change and associated health effects, and the devastating cuts at the Federal Emergency Management Agency and the Centers for Disease Control and Prevention (CDC) all point to one conclusion: we unfortunately appear on course for much more suffering from unnatural disasters.

As noted in several of the articles in this featured section, however, not only are we headed toward increased suffering, but those who will suffer most

AJPH June 2026, Vol. 116, No. 6

are likely people who are socially or economically disadvantaged. Saha et al. (p. 798) use a massive data set on emergency medical services to investigate heat-related illness and how it varies in disadvantaged or vulnerable groups. The data show that rates of use of emergency medical services for heat-related issues are higher among African Americans, Native Hawaiians/Pacific Islanders, the elderly, people living in rural areas, and those living in places classified as higher on the CDC Social Vulnerability Index than among the general population. Choa et al. (p. 779) demonstrate that lesbian, gay, bisexual, transgender, and queer (LGBTQ+) people are much more susceptible to mental health effects from disasters and housing insecurity.

Sugg et al. (p. 806) reveal how Hurricane Helene likely contributed to sustained increases in anxiety and alcohol-related emergency room use in rural areas of North Carolina, especially in elderly populations. Shannon et al. (p. 790) use a unique homeless survey to explain how virtually all people experiencing homelessness had major life disruptions or injuries from the 2025 Los Angeles wildfires. People who were completely unsheltered, however, suffered worse impacts than those who lived in shelters or vehicles. Even among an extremely disadvantaged group of people experiencing homelessness, those with the highest level of vulnerability suffered the most. Little doubt exists that climate change will endanger public health for all of us, but those most vulnerable will continue to pay the highest price. AJPH

CORRESPONDENCE

Correspondence should be sent to Michael Jerrett, PhD, 650 Charles E. Young Dr S, Room 56-070 CHS, Mail Code 177220, Los Angeles, CA 90095 (e-mail: mjerrett@ucla.edu). Reprints can be ordered at https://www.ajph.org by clicking the "Reprints" link.

PUBLICATION INFORMATION

Full Citation: Jerrett M. Public health endangerment from climate change and unnatural disasters in the Anthropocene. *Am J Public Health*. 2026;116(6): 777–778.

Acceptance Date: March 18, 2026.

DOI: https://doi.org/10.2105/AJPH.2026.308546

ORCID iD:
Michael Jerrett https://orcid.org/0000-0002-4121-0587

ACKNOWLEDGMENTS

This work was supported in part by the Jonathan Fielding Endowed Chair in Climate Change and Public Health.

CONFLICTS OF INTEREST

The author reports no conflicts of interest from funding or affiliation-related activities.

REFERENCES

1. Voosen P. The Anthropocene is dead. Long live the Anthropocene. Available at: https://www.science.org/content/article/anthropocene-dead-long-live-anthropocene. Accessed March 11, 2026.
2. Schollaert C, Connolly R, Cushing L, Jerrett M, Liu T, Marlier M. Air quality impacts of the January 2025 Los Angeles wildfires: insights from public data sources. *Environ Sci Technol Lett*. 2025;12(8): 911–917. https://doi.org/10.1021/acs.estlett.5c00486
3. Yao Y, Garcia-Gonzales D, Li J, Niu M, Nie Q, Jerrett M, Zhu Y. Indoor and outdoor volatile organic compound levels during and after the 2025 Los Angeles wildfires. *Environ Sci Technol Lett*. 2026;13(1): 70–75. https://doi.org/10.1021/acs.estlett.5c00919
4. Keeley JE, Syphard AD. Historical patterns of wildfire ignition sources in California ecosystems. *Int J Wildland Fire*. 2018;27(12):781–799. https://doi.org/10.1071/WF18026
5. National Academies of Sciences, Engineering, and Medicine. *Effects of Human-Caused Greenhouse Gas Emissions on U.S. Climate, Health, and Welfare*. Washington, DC: National Academies Press; 2025. https://doi.org/10.17226/29239
6. Greenberg M, Angelo H, Losada E, Wilmers CC. Relational geographies of urban unsustainability: the entanglement of California's housing crisis with WUI growth and climate change. *Proc Natl Acad Sci U S A*. 2024;121(32):e2310080121. https://doi.org/10.1073/pnas.2310080121
7. Hunter R, Garcia L, Dagless S, et al. The emerging syndemic of climate change and non-communicable diseases. *Lancet Planet Health*. 2024;8(7):e430–e431. https://doi.org/10.1016/s2542-5196(24)00112-8

Mental Health Disparities From Climate Change: The Role of Housing Insecurity and LGBTQ+ Identity, California, 2023

Elizabeth Choa, PhD, MSN, David Vlahov, PhD, and Hermine Poghosyan, PhD, MPH

See also Climate Change/Natural Disasters, pp. 761–813.

Objectives. To examine the relationship between housing insecurity and lesbian, gay, bisexual, pansexual, transgender, gender-expansive, queer, and questioning (LGBTQ+) identity with mental health burdens from climate events among California adults.

Methods. We used cross-sectional data from 2023 California Health Interview Survey (n = 14 307). The outcome was self-reported mental health burden from climate events. Primary predictors were LGBTQ+ identity and housing insecurity. We conducted survey-weighted descriptive statistics and multivariable logistic regression, adjusting for covariates, with an interaction term assessing synergistic effects of primary predictors.

Results. Transgender or gender-expansive (adjusted odds ratio [AOR] = 4.05; 95% confidence interval [CI] = 2.66, 6.15) and bisexual or pansexual individuals (AOR = 1.67; 95% CI = 1.19, 2.33) had significantly higher odds of climate-related mental health burden. High housing insecurity was also associated with greater odds (AOR = 1.26; 95% CI = 1.07, 1.48). Among gay respondents, experiencing housing insecurity was associated with approximately threefold higher odds of climate-related mental health burden (adjusted ratio of odds ratios = 3.1; 95% CI = 1.40, 6.82).

Conclusions. Bisexual or pansexual and transgender or gender-expansive individuals reported higher mental health burdens from climate events. Housing insecurity appears to be a key social driver shaping disparities in climate-related mental health among LGBTQ+ populations. (*Am J Public Health*. 2026;116(6): 779–789. https://doi.org/10.2105/AJPH.2025.308379)

AJPH June 2026, Vol. 116, No. 6

Climate change is an urgent public health crisis with profound effects on human health.[1] As climate events intensify, their impact extends beyond physical infrastructure and safety, increasingly threatening mental health and community well-being.[2] Exposure to these climate events has been associated with elevated levels of stress, anxiety, and trauma-related symptoms; however, the distribution of these mental health burdens is unequal.[3] Structural vulnerabilities, such as housing insecurity, play an important role in shaping who is most affected (climate vulnerability) and who can effectively recover (climate resilience).[4]

Housing stands as a key structural driver of health, exerting considerable influence on individual well-being.[5] The struggle to afford rent or meet housing costs, known as housing insecurity, is strongly linked to a range of adverse health outcomes.[6] As the largest expenditure for most households,[7] housing costs often force families to make severe trade-offs in other vital areas such as food and health care.[6] Among lower-income households, these financial constraints leave little for basic needs.[8] The ramifications of unaffordable housing extend beyond the individual and can result in financial ruin and the erosion of community bonds, both of which may worsen mental health outcomes.[5,6] Moreover, current policies and practices exacerbate these housing disparities. Changes in housing assistance policies, the targeting of nonprime loans, and ongoing housing discrimination continue to perpetuate these inequalities, further complicating the challenges faced by marginalized communities.[9,10] This issue of housing affordability is long-standing, yet the urgency of addressing it has increased as climate change escalates. In disadvantaged communities, where resources are already stretched thin, the impacts of climate change spotlight a critical area that demands comprehensive public policy responses.[11] Moreover, with the continued rise in housing costs and the increasing frequency of climate disasters, climate-driven displacement is poised to become an even more pressing challenge.[12]

Alongside housing insecurity, sexual orientation represents another often-overlooked axis of climate vulnerability. Individuals identifying as lesbian, gay, bisexual, pansexual, and queer or questioning (LGBQ+) frequently encounter a range of structural inequities, including discrimination and social exclusion, which can magnify housing challenges within these communities.[13] For instance, LGBQ+ individuals face an elevated risk of homelessness, often linked to family rejection or housing market discrimination.[14] They also face multiple vulnerabilities that can intensify health challenges, including higher rates of chronic illness, barriers to care, elevated rates of mental health challenges, and food insecurity.[15] These vulnerabilities are likely to be further amplified by climate change.

Despite these heightened risks, LGBQ+ populations remain underrepresented in climate–health research and policy.[16] Studies and policies often treat this population as homogenous, overlooking the varied health risks and needs of different subgroups within the community.[17] This lack of differentiation limits the development of nuanced policy responses. In addition, the enactment of recent anti–lesbian, gay, bisexual, pansexual, transgender, gender-expansive, queer, and questioning (LGBTQ+) policies may further impede effective public health interventions for these groups.[18] Moreover, the mental health effects of climate change, particularly at the intersection of housing insecurity and LGBQ+ identity, remain largely unexplored in population-based research.

California provides an ideal setting for this investigation. The state faces escalating climate threats, is experiencing an ongoing housing crisis, and is home to a large LGBQ+ population.[12] This backdrop is suitable for exploring how these factors converge to influence climate-related mental health burdens. By focusing on populations often underrepresented in climate–health research, this study examines the relationship between housing insecurity, LGBQ+ identity, and mental health burdens from climate events.

METHODS

In this study, we analyzed cross-sectional data from the 2023 California Health Interview Survey (CHIS), the largest statewide population health survey in the country. CHIS employs a complex address-based sampling design to generate representative estimates of California's noninstitutionalized adult population. Full methodological details are available in CHIS technical reports.[19] In 2023, a total of 21 671 individuals were interviewed. Among these, 14 319 self-reported exposure to a hazardous climate event. After excluding 12 proxy respondents with missing values from a reduced questionnaire, the final analytic sample comprised 14 307 individuals. All data are self-reported. Data collection spanned from January to December 2023.[19]

Mental Health Burden From Climate Change

The dichotomous (yes, no) outcome variable was negative mental health impacts from climate events, measured using a series of multipart questions. All respondents were first asked, "In the past two years, have you [or members of your household] personally experienced: Extreme heat wave? Wildfire? Smoke from wildfire? Flood/rising sea levels/mudslide?" Those who responded "yes" to any of these received the follow-up question: "Was your mental health [or the mental health of members of your household] harmed by any of these events?" Participants who responded affirmatively were classified as having experienced adverse climate-related mental health impacts.

Housing Insecurity and Sexual Orientation

Housing insecurity and LGBQ+ identity were the primary predictors. Housing insecurity was measured by how frequently respondents worried about affording rent or mortgage. Those reporting concerns "somewhat often" or "very often" were classified as experiencing high housing insecurity.

LGBQ+ identity was based on survey responses to sexual orientation, with options including lesbian or gay, and bisexual or pansexual. Responses such as "I use a different term," "Don't know," and "Prefer not to answer" were grouped as "other" to capture the broader spectrum of queer+ identities, including those questioning, exploring, or withholding their identities. For detailed analyses, we disaggregated the category "Lesbian or Gay" by assigned sex at birth. Respondents assigned male who identified as "Lesbian or Gay" were categorized as gay, and those assigned female as lesbian. In this study, sexual orientation refers to all reported categories, including straight, while LGBQ+ identity refers specifically to nonheterosexual orientations. It is important to note that sexual orientation differs fundamentally from gender identity (e.g., transgender or gender-expansive), though both are often combined under the LGBTQ+ acronym. In our analyses, sexual orientation was treated as the primary predictor, with transgender or gender-expansive identity included as a covariate.

Covariates

We selected predictors that have been previously reported as relevant to mental health,[20,21] including age (18–29, 30–39, 40–49, 50–64, 65–74, ≥ 75 years), race/ethnicity (Hispanic, non-Hispanic White, non-Hispanic Black, non-Hispanic Asian, other or 2 or more races), educational attainment (high-school graduate or less, vocational school/associate's degree/some college, college graduate or more), employment status (full, part time, unemployed), household income (< 200% federal poverty level, ≥ 200% federal poverty level, based on US Department of Health and Human Services guidelines), marital status (never married, married/living with partner, widowed/separated/divorced), general health status (poor/fair, good, very good/excellent), and psychological distress in the past year (yes, no). We also included covariates that are less studied in the context of climate–mental health, including assigned sex at birth (female, male), transgender identity (transgender/gender expansive, cisgender/gender-conforming), housing situation (homeowner in a single-unit building, renting in a multiunit building, renting in a single-unit building, homeowner in a multiunit building, living with other arrangements), rurality (urban, rural), and community cohesion, which was measured based on willingness to help neighbors (strongly disagree/disagree, agree/strongly agree).

Statistical Analysis

We employed a range of analytic methods, beginning with descriptive analyses to summarize sample characteristics, including unweighted counts and weighted proportions. We used descriptive statistics, cross-tabulation analysis, and the Wald χ^2 test to assess variations in the distribution of factors by adverse mental health impacts from climate events, housing insecurity, and LGBQ+ identity. We then fit a weighted multivariable logistic regression model to examine the impact of LGBQ+ identity and housing insecurity on climate-related mental health impacts, adjusting for covariates. We quantified associations using odds ratios (ORs) and 95% confidence intervals (CIs). In addition, we included interaction terms along with the main effects to examine whether the synergistic effects of housing insecurity and LGBQ+ identity differed from their individual effects. We used joint significance tests to evaluate whether categorical variables and interaction terms contributed meaningfully to the overall model. We conducted all analyses in Stata version 18 (StataCorp LP, College Station, TX). We applied sampling weights to account for the complex survey design, with the jackknife method used for variance estimation.[22]

RESULTS

Descriptive characteristics of the weighted sample population (n = 17 861 613 adults) are available in Table A (available as a supplement to the online version of this article at https://ajph.org). Among adults who experienced a climate event, 23.4% were aged 18 to 29 years, 34.9% were Hispanic, 50.8% were assigned female at birth, and 42.0% reported high housing insecurity. Overall, 23.5% of study participants reported having their mental health harmed by climate events.

The analysis identified significant disparities associated with high housing insecurity ($P < .001$). Respondents facing high housing insecurity demonstrated a higher prevalence of adverse mental health impacts from climate events (27.8%) than those with more housing security (20.4%) ($P < .001$). Similarly, we observed significant differences in outcomes across sexual orientations and transgender identity (both $P < .001$). Bisexual or pansexual respondents reported the highest prevalence of adverse mental health impacts (49.2%) compared with straight respondents (21.5%; $P < .001$). In addition, transgender or gender-expansive individuals had a higher prevalence of negative mental health impacts related to climate events (63.4%) compared with cisgender individuals (22.8%; $P < .001$).

Sample Characteristics

Table 1 presents the distribution of characteristics by housing insecurity and LGBQ+ identity. The proportion of respondents experiencing high housing insecurity was greater among younger adults (26.4% for those aged 18 to 29 years vs 8.0% for those aged 65 to 74 years; $P < .001$), homeowners in a single-unit building (41.0% vs 16.6% for

AJPH June 2026, Vol. 116, No. 6

TABLE 1— Weighted Descriptive Summary of Adults Who Experienced a Climate Event by Housing Insecurity and LGBQ+ Identity: 2023 California Health Interview Survey

	Low Housing Insecurity (n = 8874), Weighted % (95% CI)	High Housing Insecurity (n = 5433), Weighted % (95% CI)	P	Lesbian (n = 205), Weighted % (95% CI)	Gay (n = 357), Weighted % (95% CI)	Bisexual or Pansexual (n = 704), Weighted % (95% CI)	Other (n = 625), Weighted % (95% CI)	P
Age group, y			< .001					< .001
18–29	21.1 (20.0, 22.4)	26.4 (24.9, 28.1)		38.5 (30.4, 47.5)	19.0 (14.0, 25.2)	59.6 (54.3, 64.6)	32.6 (27.6, 38.0)	
30–39	15.4 (14.5, 16.5)	20.9 (19.7, 22.1)		17.5 (12.1, 24.5)	23.9 (18.0, 31.2)	20.5 (16.9, 24.8)	14.7 (11.2, 19.2)	
40–49	13.8 (12.9, 14.7)	18.5 (17.4, 19.6)		10.8 (5.7, 19.4)	21.3 (15.4, 28.8)	8.7 (6.7, 11.3)	15.7 (12.8, 19.0)	
50–64	22.6 (21.6, 23.6)	22.2 (20.8, 23.6)		20.1 (14.1, 28.0)	20.9 (16.3, 26.5)	7.3 (5.5, 9.7)	16.6 (12.7, 21.4)	
65–74	16.5 (15.6, 17.4)	8.0 (7.2, 9.0)		7.3 (4.9, 10.8)	10.3 (7.0, 17.8)	3.0 (2.0, 4.4)	15.1 (11.9, 18.9)	
≥75	10.6 (9.9, 11.3)	4.0 (3.4, 4.6)		5.8 (3.5, 9.3)	4.6 (2.7, 7.7)	0.9 (0.5, 1.4)	5.3 (3.6, 7.8)	
Race/ethnicity			< .001					< .001
Non-Hispanic White	51.7 (50.5, 52.8)	33.5 (32.0, 35.2)		61.1 (51.0, 70.3)	54.0 (46.2, 61.6)	38.3 (33.8, 43.1)	30.5 (25.9, 35.6)	
Hispanic	27.7 (26.5, 29.0)	44.8 (43.0, 46.6)		23.3 (16.1, 32.4)	28.2 (22.1, 35.3)	42.9 (37.9, 48.0)	42.4 (36.3, 48.7)	
Non-Hispanic African American	4.6 (4.1, 5.2)	5.1 (4.4, 6.0)		5.9 (3.1, 11.2)	3.5 (1.3, 9.3)	2.1 (0.7, 5.6)	3.3 (2.3, 4.8)	
Non-Hispanic Asian	13.1 (12.3, 14.0)	13.8 (12.7, 15.1)		4.4 (1.7, 10.7)	12.1 (7.6, 18.7)	12.2 (9.0, 16.5)	20.7 (16.2, 26.0)	
Other or 2 or more races/ethnicities	2.9 (2.6, 3.3)	2.8 (2.3, 3.3)		5.3 (1.9, 13.8)	2.2 (1.1, 4.5)	4.5 (3.0, 6.7)	3.1 (1.7, 5.6)	
Educational attainment			< .001					< .001
High school or less	27.7 (26.4, 29.0)	36.7 (35.0, 38.4)		23.7 (17.0, 32.0)	21.2 (14.9, 29.1)	25.9 (21.8, 30.5)	53.6 (48.2, 59.0)	
Some college or vocational	19.4 (18.4, 20.5)	23.7 (22.1, 25.3)		21.3 (15.0, 29.4)	20.1 (15.1, 26.3)	22.1 (18.5, 26.1)	15.5 (12.5, 19.1)	
College or higher	52.9 (51.6, 54.2)	39.6 (38.0, 41.3)		55.0 (45.9, 63.8)	58.7 (51.0, 66.1)	52.0 (47.1, 57.0)	30.9 (26.6, 35.4)	
Marital status			< .001					< .001
Never married	25.9 (24.5, 27.3)	30.6 (28.8, 32.4)		43.6 (34.3, 53.3)	49.5 (41.9, 57.1)	54.5 (49.8, 59.2)	44.1 (39.1, 49.3)	
Married or living with partner	60.9 (59.5, 62.3)	55.1 (53.1, 57.0)		50.5 (41.6, 59.4)	45.2 (37.9, 52.7)	40.5 (36.1, 45.1)	45.4 (41.1, 49.8)	
Widow, separated, or divorced	13.2 (12.3, 14.1)	14.3 (13.2, 15.6)		5.9 (3.5, 9.7)	5.3 (3.2, 8.6)	5.0 (3.6, 6.7)	10.5 (8.2, 13.2)	
Sex assigned at birth			.07					< .001
Male	50.1 (48.9, 51.4)	47.9 (46.5, 49.4)		0	100	34.0 (29.7, 38.7)	42.5 (37.0, 48.1)	
Female	49.9 (48.6, 51.1)	52.1 (50.6, 53.5)		100	0	66.0 (61.3, 70.3)	57.5 (51.9, 63.0)	
Sexual orientation			< .001					. . .
Straight	85.2 (84.1, 86.4)	81.3 (80.0, 82.6)		. . .	. . .	. . .	. . .	
Lesbian	1.2 (0.9, 1.5)	1.4 (1.2, 1.8)		. . .	. . .	. . .	. . .	
Gay	2.8 (2.4, 3.2)	2.2 (1.7, 2.8)		. . .	. . .	. . .	. . .	
Bisexual or pansexual	5.2 (4.5, 6.0)	8.4 (7.3, 9.5)		. . .	. . .	. . .	. . .	
Other	5.6 (4.9, 6.4)	6.7 (5.7, 7.7)		. . .	. . .	. . .	. . .	
Transgender identity			.17					< .001
Cisgender	98.4 (98.0, 98.8)	98.0 (97.4, 98.4)		82.8 (77.6, 87.0)	93.0 (89.3, 95.5)	88.8 (84.7, 91.9)	92.0 (89.6, 93.9)	

Continued

TABLE 1— Continued

	Low Housing Insecurity (n = 8874), Weighted % (95% CI)	High Housing Insecurity (n = 5433), Weighted % (95% CI)	P	Lesbian (n = 205), Weighted % (95% CI)	Gay (n = 357), Weighted % (95% CI)	Bisexual or Pansexual (n = 704), Weighted % (95% CI)	Other (n = 625), Weighted % (95% CI)	P
Trans or gender expansive	1.6 (1.2, 2.0)	2.0 (1.6, 2.6)		17.2 (13.0, 22.5)	7.0 (4.5, 10.8)	11.2 (8.1, 15.3)	8.0 (6.1, 10.5)	
Employment			< .001					< .001
Full time, ≥ 21 h per week	52.2 (50.7, 53.6)	58.5 (56.8, 60.1)		62.8 (55.0, 70.0)	69.1 (62.3, 75.2)	59.0 (53.6, 64.3)	42.9 (38.0, 48.0)	
Part time, 0–20 h per week	8.4 (7.5, 9.4)	9.6 (8.6, 10.8)		13.2 (8.1, 20.8)	4.7 (2.9, 7.3)	12.1 (9.3, 15.5)	13.1 (10.1, 16.8)	
Unemployed	39.4 (38.0, 40.9)	31.9 (30.3, 33.6)		24.0 (18.2, 31.0)	26.2 (20.7, 32.7)	28.9 (24.4, 33.8)	44.0 (38.4, 49.7)	
Household income			< .001					< .001
< 200% FPL	19.3 (18.0, 20.8)	36.8 (35.0, 38.7)		13.5 (9.2, 19.5)	16.6 (11.4, 23.5)	27.0 (23.2, 31.1)	45.3 (40.0, 50.7)	
≥ 200% FPL	80.7 (79.2, 82.0)	63.2 (61.3, 65.0)		86.5 (80.5, 90.8)	83.4 (76.5, 88.6)	73.0 (68.9, 76.8)	54.7(49.3, 60.0)	
General health			< .001					< .001
Fair–poor	12.6 (11.5, 13.8)	22.8 (21.0, 24.7)		15.2 (9.8, 22.8)	9.0 (5.9, 13.4)	20.4 (17.1, 24.0)	32.0 (26.7, 37.8)	
Good	29.7 (28.3, 31.2)	35.4 (33.3, 37.6)		29.5 (22.1, 38.2)	31.8 (25.5, 38.8)	32.0 (28.1, 36.2)	34.4 (29.0, 40.3)	
Excellent–very good	57.7 (56.2, 59.2)	41.8 (39.7, 43.8)		55.4 (46.5, 63.9)	59.3 (51.8, 66.3)	47.6 (43.2, 52.1)	33.6 (28.7, 38.7)	
Psychological distress			< .001					< .001
None in last year	89.6 (88.7, 90.5)	74.0 (72.1, 75.9)		81.3 (75.6, 87.7)	79.3 (71.6, 85.3)	47.1 (52.5, 51.8)	76.5 (71.4, 80.9)	
Yes in last year	10.4 (9.5, 11.3)	26.0 (24.1, 27.9)		18.7 (12.3, 27.4)	20.7 (14.7, 28.4)	52.9 (48.2, 57.5)	23.5 (19.1, 28.7)	
Rurality			< .001					.001
Urban	85.8 (85.0, 86.6)	89.5 (88.3, 90.6)		92.8 (86.9, 96.2)	90.3 (86.6, 93.1)	90.9 (87.3, 93.6)	90.0 (86.4, 92.7)	
Rural	14.2 (13.4, 15.0)	10.5 (9.4, 11.7)		7.2 (3.8, 13.1)	9.7 (6.9, 13.4)	9.1 (6.4, 12.7)	10.0 (7.3, 13.6)	
Housing insecurity								< .001
Low	. . .	. . .		52.9 (44.9, 60.9)	63.4 (55.8, 70.4)	46.1 (40.8, 51.5)	53.7 (48.2, 59.0)	
High	. . .	. . .		47.1 (39.1, 55.1)	36.6 (29.6, 44.2)	53.9 (48.5, 59.2)	46.3 (41.0, 51.8)	
Housing situation			< .001					< .001
Homeowner single-unit building	64.0 (62.5, 65.5)	41.0 (39.3, 42.9)		46.6 (38.0, 55.5)	43.2 (35.8, 51.0)	34.2 (29.8, 38.9)	42.6 (36.8, 48.7)	
Renting multi-unit building	16.5 (15.3, 17.7)	31.2 (29.7, 32.7)		33.2 (26.0, 41.3)	34.6 (27.9, 42.0)	37.7 (33.0, 42.8)	25.2 (20.6, 30.6)	
Renting single-unit building	7.3 (6.5, 8.3)	16.6 (15.1, 18.3		5.7 (3.0, 10.3)	7.5 (4.6, 12.0)	15.8 (12.3, 20.1)	14.7 (10.7, 19.8)	
Homeowner multi-unit building	6.9 (6.2, 7.7)	5.6 (4.7, 6.5)		10.0 (5.6, 17.4)	12.1 (7.6, 18.6)	4.3 (2.8, 6.4)	8.3 (5.2, 12.8)	
Living other arrangement	5.3 (4.6, 6.0)	5.6 (4.6, 6.7)		4.5 (2.3, 8.6)	2.6 (0.9, 7.2)	8.0 (5.3, 11.9)	9.2 (7.1, 11.8)	
Community cohesion			< .001					< .001
High	87.1 (86.0, 88.1)	75.2 (73.6, 76.8)		87.4 (81.5, 91.7)	74.7 (66.6, 81.4)	73.4 (68.5, 77.8)	80.9 (75.9, 85.0)	
Low	12.9 (11.9, 14.0)	24.8 (23.2, 26.4)		12.6 (8.3, 18.5)	25.3 (18.6, 33.4)	26.6 (22.2, 31.5)	19.1 (15.0, 24.1)	

Note. CI = confidence interval; FPL = federal poverty level (based on US Department of Health and Human Services guidelines); LGBQ+ = lesbian, gay, bisexual, pansexual, and queer or questioning. Sample sizes are unweighted. *P* values derived from χ^2 test.

renters in a single-unit building; $P<.001$), and urban residents (89.5% vs 10.5% for rural; $P<.001$). Urban residency was more common among all LGBQ+ respondents, with lesbian individuals showing the highest proportion at 92.8% ($P=.001$). Bisexual or pansexual individuals also recorded the highest proportion among LGBQ+ in several categories: they were predominantly younger (59.6% aged 18 to 29 years), experienced the highest proportion of psychological distress (52.9%), experienced high housing insecurity (53.9%), and lived in neighborhoods with low community cohesion (26.6%; all $P<.001$). Within other LGBQ+ groups, gay individuals (25.3%) were the next largest proportion of respondents living in neighborhoods with low community cohesion. Lesbians had the highest proportion living in neighborhoods with high community cohesion (87.4%; $P<.001$).

Multivariable Analysis

Table 2 presents the results from multivariable analyses. Odds of reporting adverse mental health impacts from climate events were lower with age (50 to 64 years: AOR = 0.72; 95% CI = 0.58, 0.90; ≥ 75 years: AOR = 0.53; 95% CI = 0.38, 0.75; vs 18 to 29 years). Hispanic (AOR = 0.60; 95% CI = 0.51, 0.71) and Asian adults (AOR = 0.55; 95% CI = 0.46, 0.66) also had lower odds than White adults. By contrast, transgender or gender-expansive adults had approximately 4 times the odds of cisgender adults (AOR = 4.05; 95% CI = 2.66, 6.15).

Sexual orientation was associated with a similar overall pattern across groups, with associations attenuating toward the null after adjustment. For example, lesbian adults with low housing insecurity had an unadjusted odds ratio of 1.63 (95% CI = 1.17, 2.26), which was not statistically significant after adjustment (AOR = 0.78; 95% CI = 0.44, 1.39). By contrast, bisexual or pansexual adults with low housing insecurity remained at significantly higher risk compared with straight adults (AOR = 1.67; 95% CI = 1.19, 2.33). Straight individuals with high housing insecurity had greater odds of climate-related mental health burdens than those with low insecurity (AOR = 1.26; 95% CI = 1.07, 1.48). AORs for housing insecurity by LGBQ+ identity and corresponding unweighted sample sizes are shown in Table B (available as a supplement to the online version of this article at https://ajph.org).

Results for housing and community context factors indicated that renters in multiunit buildings had lower odds compared with single-unit homeowners (AOR = 0.82; 95% CI = 0.68, 0.97), whereas owners in multiunit buildings had higher odds (AOR = 1.34; 95% CI = 1.02, 1.77). Residents of neighborhoods with low community cohesion and those in rural areas also had higher odds of climate-related mental health impacts (AOR = 1.29; 95% CI = 1.08, 1.54; AOR = 1.53; 95% CI = 1.33, 1.77, respectively).

The interaction term of housing insecurity and LGBQ+ identity on climate-related mental health burdens was statistically significant. Specifically, gay respondents experiencing housing insecurity had approximately threefold increase in the odds of reporting adverse mental health impacts from climate events (adjusted ratio of odds ratios [AROR] = 3.1; 95% CI = 1.40, 6.82). Bisexual or pansexual respondents experiencing housing insecurity also had elevated odds, though less pronounced (AROR = 1.59; 95% CI = 0.98, 2.57).

DISCUSSION

The study findings suggest climate-related mental health disparities among housing insecure and LGBQ+ populations.

Demographic Factors

The patterns observed in our study challenge several commonly held assumptions about vulnerability to climate–health impacts. While it is often reported that racial and ethnic minority individuals and older populations are more susceptible to adverse health effects of climate change,[23] our findings indicate the potential for greater climate-related mental health resilience within these communities.

One possible explanation for this finding among racial and ethnic minority individuals is that experiencing discrimination or structural racism may contribute to the development of adaptive strategies.[24] These strategies could support mental resilience, enabling individuals to more effectively manage climate-related stressors. This does not suggest immunity to distress but, rather, emphasizes the importance of recognizing varied responses and exploring protective factors that may positively influence mental well-being in the context of climate change. Similarly, our findings indicate lower odds of reporting climate-related mental health impacts among older adults, which diverges from previous research identifying older populations as particularly vulnerable.[25] The reasons for this discrepancy are unclear but may relate to differences in accumulated life experiences, levels of social support, or perceived time horizons for climate threats. Together, these findings challenge prevailing narratives about vulnerability and

TABLE 2— Weighted Multivariable Logistic Regression of Housing Insecurity, LGBQ+ Identity, and Climate-Related Mental Health Harm Among Adults Who Experienced a Climate Event: 2023 California Health Interview Survey

Characteristics	Simple Logistic Regressions,[a] OR (95% CI) or *P*	Multivariable Logistic Regression, AOR (95% CI)
Age group, y	<.001	<.001
18–29 (Ref)	1	1
30–39	1.12 (0.90, 1.39)	1.07 (0.84, 1.38)
40–49	0.75 (0.62, 0.90)	0.81 (0.64, 1.00)
50–64	0.65 (0.56, 0.76)	0.72 (0.58, 0.90)
65–74	0.59 (0.49, 0.71)	0.64 (0.49, 0.84)
≥75	0.50 (0.39, 0.63)	0.53 (0.38, 0.75)
Race/ethnicity	<.001	<.001
Non-Hispanic White (Ref)	1	1
Hispanic	0.68 (0.59, 0.78)	0.60 (0.51, 0.71)
Non-Hispanic African American	0.72 (0.50, 1.02)	0.76 (0.53, 1.08)
Non-Hispanic Asian	0.66 (0.56, 0.78)	0.55 (0.46, 0.66)
Other or 2 or more races/ethnicities	1.09 (0.82, 1.43)	0.99 (0.73, 1.36)
Educational attainment	<.001	<.001
High school or less (Ref)	1	1
Some college or vocational	1.42 (1.21, 1.67)	1.29 (1.09, 1.53)
College or higher	1.65 (1.40, 1.94)	1.63 (1.36, 1.96)
Marital status	.002	.01
Never married (Ref)	1	1
Married or living with partner	0.95 (0.82, 1.09)	1.33 (1.10, 1.61)
Widow, separated, or divorced	0.72 (0.59, 0.86)	1.13 (0.91, 1.41)
Sex assigned at birth	<.001	.006
Male (Ref)	1	1
Female	1.26 (1.12, 1.43)	1.18 (1.05, 1.34)
Sexual orientation	<.001	<.001
Straight (Ref)	1	1
Lesbian	1.63 (1.17, 2.26)	0.78 (0.44, 1.39)
Gay	1.45 (1.05, 2.01)	0.79 (0.50, 1.24)
Bisexual or pansexual	3.54 (2.92, 4.28)	1.67 (1.19, 2.33)
Other	0.97 (0.76, 1.23)	0.76 (0.52, 1.12)
Transgender identity	<.001	<.001
Cisgender (Ref)	1	1
Transgender or gender expansive	5.86 (4.21, 8.17)	4.05 (2.66, 6.15)
Employment status	.025	.86
Full time, ≥21 h per week (Ref)	1	1
Part time, 0–20 h per week	0.90 (0.75, 1.07)	0.97 (0.79, 1.18)
Unemployed	0.85 (0.76, 0.96)	1.03 (0.88, 1.20)
Household income	.42	.17
<200% FPL (Ref)	1	1
≥200% FPL	1.05 (0.93, 1.18)	0.90 (0.77, 1.04)
General health	.039	.037
Fair–poor (Ref)	1	1

Continued

TABLE 2— Continued

Characteristics	Simple Logistic Regressions,[a] OR (95% CI) or P	Multivariable Logistic Regression, AOR (95% CI)
Good	0.90 (0.76, 1.07)	0.88 (0.74, 1.04)
Excellent–very good	0.85 (0.75, 0.96)	0.82 (0.70, 0.95)
Psychological distress	<.001	<.001
None in last year (Ref)	1	1
Yes in last year	3.15 (2.76, 3.59)	2.38 (2.03, 2.79)
Rurality	<.001	<.001
Urban (Ref)	1	1
Rural	1.37 (1.21, 1.56)	1.53 (1.33, 1.77)
Housing insecurity	<.001	<.001
Low (Ref)	1	1
High	1.50 (1.33, 1.70)	1.26 (1.07, 1.48)
Housing situation	.08	.053
Homeowner single-unit building (Ref)	1	1
Renting multi-unit building	1.13 (1.00, 1.27)	0.82 (0.68, 0.97)
Renting single-unit building	1.19 (0.95, 1.49)	0.97 (0.74, 1.24)
Homeowner multi-unit building	1.30 (1.01, 1.66)	1.34 (1.02, 1.77)
Living with other arrangements	1.00 (0.73, 1.37)	0.85 (0.59, 1.23)
Community cohesion	<.001	.006
High (Ref)	1	1
Low	1.41 (1.21, 1.64)	1.29 (1.08, 1.54)
High housing insecurity * LGBQ+ identity (ratio of ORs)	.024	.024
High housing insecurity * lesbian (n = 97)	2.69 (1.68, 4.32)	1.70 (0.81, 3.58)
High housing insecurity * gay (n = 130)	3.48 (2.01, 6.02)	3.10 (1.40, 6.82)
High housing insecurity * bisexual/pansexual (n = 365)	5.63 (4.40, 7.21)	1.59 (0.98, 2.57)
High housing insecurity * other (n = 625)	1.27 (0.92, 1.76)	1.18 (0.67, 2.09)

Note. AOR = adjusted odds ratio; CI = confidence interval; FPL = federal poverty level (based on US Department of Health and Human Services guidelines); LGBQ+ = lesbian, gay, bisexual, pansexual, and queer or questioning; OR = odds ratio. Sexual orientation includes all categories (straight as reference), whereas LGBQ+ identity is used for interaction term to denote nonheterosexual identities. Total unweighted sample = 14 307. Total weighted sample = 17 861 613.

[a]Results show outcomes from individual logistic regressions with separate models for each predictor. For interaction terms, the main effects were included in the simple logistic regressions.

highlight the importance of considering protective factors and sources of resilience in our understanding of how different populations respond to climate challenges.

Housing Factors

Our findings highlight how housing context may shape mental health impacts from climate events. While previous research portrays renters as more vulnerable to climate-related health impacts,[26] we identified a counterintuitive pattern: homeowners in single-unit buildings reported greater odds of mental health burdens from climate events than did renters in multiunit buildings. This unexpected finding may reflect the financial strains and psychological stresses of homeownership intensifying under the pressures of climate change. Homeowners face the risk of property damage and the need for substantial financial investments to mitigate climate threats, such as reinforcing homes or acquiring additional insurance.[27] With climate disasters increasing, shifts in the mortgage and insurance markets could lead to reduced coverage or higher premiums in high-risk areas like California, adding further instability for homeowners.[28] Traditionally considered a stable investment, homeownership has become increasingly associated with layers of vulnerability amid growing climate threats.

By contrast, renters in multiunit buildings may benefit from flexibility and smaller financial commitments to any single property. Their capacity to relocate more readily in response to climate threats, combined with fewer long-term financial obligations tied to their housing situation, may help cushion some of the mental health burdens from climate events. This relative mobility may confer an adaptive advantage less accessible to homeowners, highlighting a shift in how different housing arrangements shape mental health burdens in the context of climate change.

Sexual Orientation and Gender Diversity

To better capture the diversity within LGBQ+ communities and address the underrepresentation of bisexual individuals in research,[29] we disaggregated responses from bisexual or pansexual, lesbian, and gay participants. This approach was a strength of our study as it allowed us to identify group-specific vulnerabilities often obscured in broader categorizations.

Bisexual or pansexual individuals, as well as those identifying as transgender or gender-expansive, had higher odds of mental health burdens related to climate events. For transgender and gender-expansive respondents, the odds were especially elevated (AOR = 4.05; 95% CI = 2.66, 6.15). Although the relatively small sample size (n = 152) warrants cautious interpretation, its consistency with broader literature supports the importance of this finding and indicates that larger studies should be prioritized to strengthen the evidence base.

Both bisexual or pansexual and transgender or gender-expansive groups defy traditional binary norms, which may heighten exposure to discrimination and social exclusion.[30] Such marginalization could contribute to greater susceptibility to mental health challenges, especially following climate events. These risks appear more severe when emergency and recovery services, including shelters and medical clinics, fail to offer inclusive environments. Shelters and clinics, often managed by organizations without affirming care practices, have been documented to deny assistance to sexual and gender minority people.[31] The elevated rates observed in these groups call for research that reflects their distinct circumstances and for policies that ensure access to safe and responsive systems of care.

Our results support existing literature that documents an increase in bisexual identification among young adults.[29] This trend may reflect a shift in cultural norms and enhanced visibility of bisexuality; however, despite this greater recognition, bisexual people continue to face distinct health challenges, such as lower societal acceptance and dual discrimination from both heterosexual and LGBQ+ communities.[32] This pattern of increased bisexual identification is consistent with our observation that young adults appeared more likely to report mental health burdens from climate events, possibly because of a mix of age-related and identity-specific stressors.

Our analysis also introduced interaction terms to explore compound risks. Notably, we observed that the combination of gay identity and high housing insecurity together was associated with higher odds of mental health burdens from climate events, more than either factor independently. This finding is compelling given the broader societal acceptance of gay and lesbian identities in recent years. The increased risk may be related to patterns of antigay prejudice rooted in gender-role ideologies that more harshly penalize male femininity.[33] Since gay men are commonly stereotyped as feminine, studies suggest they may face greater stigma and negative perceptions than lesbians.[34] Furthermore, recent anti-LGBTQ+ legislation in the United States appears to be intensifying this discrimination,[35] potentially limiting access to critical resources such as employment, housing, and social capital.[34] For gay people experiencing high housing insecurity, these compounded stressors could undermine their capacity to manage mental health challenges posed by climate events. More broadly, this finding highlights the complexity of contemporary attitudes toward LGBTQ+ rights, which, despite increasing societal acceptance, continue to operate within systems shaped by heterosexual norms and privilege. Further research is needed to clarify how sexual orientation, gender identity, and housing instability interact to shape mental health in the context of climate change.

Limitations

This study has several limitations. Reliance on self-reported data introduces subjectivity, though it remains a well-established method for capturing perceived harm and subclinical impacts in mental health research. The absence of objective climate exposure measures and use of a combined indicator spanning multiple event types may introduce heterogeneity, pointing to the need for future work integrating localized climate data with survey responses. Item wording may also have led respondents in multiperson households to consider others' experiences, raising the possibility of ecological fallacy.

Survey design further constrained interpretation. Sexual orientation and

AJPH June 2026, Vol. 116, No. 6

gender identity were captured with limited categories, and grouping some responses into "other" may have introduced misclassification. The small subsample of transgender and gender-expansive respondents (n = 152) produced a large AOR (4.05), which should be interpreted cautiously given the wide confidence interval. While consistent with previous literature, a fuller analysis of gender identity as a primary predictor was beyond this study's scope. Finally, because the survey was conducted in California and excluded individuals experiencing unsheltered or hidden forms of homelessness, findings may have limited generalizability and may not fully capture the burden among the most housing-insecure populations.

Public Health Implications

This study provides valuable insights into the mental health burdens of climate events, with a focus on housing-insecure and LGBQ+ populations. Few studies have examined these challenges through the dual perspectives of housing insecurity and LGBQ+ identity, 2 drivers of health that remain underexamined in climate–health research. The findings point to the need for more inclusive frameworks in climate adaptation planning and mental health response systems. Addressing either housing insecurity or LGBQ+ disparities in isolation overlooks the layered vulnerabilities that shape individual experiences. Coordinated, multisectoral efforts are essential, integrating stable housing, accessible and inclusive mental health care, and targeted outreach to LGBQ+ communities within broader climate resilience strategies. Equally important are investments in social cohesion and mutual aid networks, which can buffer psychological harm during and after climate events. At the policy level, embedding protections for housing-insecure and LGBQ+ populations into disaster preparedness and recovery can help ensure adaptation measures reach those most at risk. Together, these directions demonstrate how multilevel strategies can advance public health action and strengthen resilience in practice.

A key contribution of this study is its examination of findings across distinct LGBTQ+ groups. Results indicated greater susceptibility of bisexual or pansexual and transgender or gender-expansive people to adverse mental health impacts from climate events. The combination of gay identity and high housing insecurity was also associated with higher odds of climate-related mental health impacts than either factor alone, highlighting the complex interplay between housing, LGBQ+ identity, and mental health. These findings call for more extensive climate–health research and policies that directly address these disparities, as well as strategies to strengthen climate resilience within these populations.

Finally, without targeted and sustained action, climate change may exacerbate health inequities among many marginalized groups. Addressing these disparities demands continuous equity-focused research across disciplines, the enactment of protective legislation, and genuine collaboration with impacted communities. Prioritizing the protection of the most vulnerable populations should remain a central focus in public health and policy. This commitment is not only vital for those most at risk but also essential for maintaining the health and resilience of all communities in the face of climate change. AJPH

ABOUT THE AUTHORS

Elizabeth Choa was with the Graduate School of Arts and Sciences and School of Nursing, Yale University, New Haven, CT, at the time of this study. David Vlahov is with the School of Nursing and the School of Public Health, Yale University. Hermine Poghosyan is with the School of Nursing, Yale University.

CORRESPONDENCE

Correspondence should be sent to Elizabeth Choa, 1100 Glendon Ave, Suite 900, Los Angeles, CA 90024 (e-mail: echoa@mednet.ucla.edu). Reprints can be ordered at https://www.ajph.org by clicking the "Reprints" link.

PUBLICATION INFORMATION

Full Citation: Choa E, Vlahov D, Poghosyan H. Mental health disparities from climate change: the role of housing insecurity and LGBTQ+ identity, California, 2023. *Am J Public Health*. 2026;116(6): 779–789.

Acceptance Date: November 28, 2025.

DOI: https://doi.org/10.2105/AJPH.2025.308379

ORCID iDs:

Elizabeth Choa https://orcid.org/0000-0003-1813-910X

David Vlahov https://orcid.org/0000-0002-3449-8068

CONTRIBUTORS

E. Choa originated and designed the study, led the data analysis and interpretation, and drafted the article, overseeing its revision. D. Vlahov contributed meaningfully to the study design, data analysis and interpretation, and article drafting, with substantial input through revision. H. Poghosyan oversaw the data analysis and interpretation, contributed to the study design, and revised the article for important intellectual content. All authors approved the final version and agree to be accountable for all aspects of the work.

ACKNOWLEDGMENTS

The authors gratefully acknowledge the UCLA Center for Health Policy Research for providing access to the California Health Interview Survey (CHIS) data. Sincere thanks are also extended to Sayantani Sarkar for her mentorship during the early stages of the analysis and to David Weitzenkamp for his technical guidance throughout the development of this work. The authors also acknowledge support provided to E. Choa by the UCLA National Clinician Scholars Program and David Eisenman during article revisions.

CONFLICTS OF INTEREST

The authors report no conflicts of interest.

HUMAN PARTICIPANT PROTECTION

This study was determined to be exempt by the Yale University institutional review board because it involved secondary analysis of publicly available data.

CHIS maintains a rigorous informed consent process emphasizing voluntary participation and confidentiality.

REFERENCES

1. World Health Organization. *COP26 Special Report on Climate Change and Health: The Health Argument for Climate Action.* 2021. Available at: https://iris.who.int/handle/10665/346168. Accessed April 3, 2025.
2. Berry HL, Waite TD, Dear KB, Capon AG, Murray V. The case for systems thinking about climate change and mental health. *Nature Clim Change.* 2018;8(4):282–290. https://doi.org/10.1038/s41558-018-0102-4
3. Cianconi P, Betrò S, Janiri L. The impact of climate change on mental health: a systematic descriptive review. *Front Psychiatry.* 2020;11:74. https://doi.org/10.3389/fpsyt.2020.00074
4. Thomas K, Hardy RD, Lazrus H, et al. Explaining differential vulnerability to climate change: a social science review. *Wiley Interdiscip Rev Clim Change.* 2019;10(2):e565. https://doi.org/10.1002/wcc.565
5. Swope CB, Hernández D. Housing as a determinant of health equity: a conceptual model. *Soc Sci Med.* 2019;243:112571. https://doi.org/10.1016/j.socscimed.2019.112571
6. DeLuca S, Rosen E. Housing insecurity among the poor today. *Annu Rev Sociol.* 2022;48(1):343–371. https://doi.org/10.1146/annurev-soc-090921-040646
7. US Bureau of Labor Statistics. *Consumer Expenditures in 2020.* Washington, DC: US Department of Labor; 2021.
8. Airgood-Obrycki W, Hermann A, Wedeen S. "The rent eats first": rental housing unaffordability in the United States. *Hous Policy Debate.* 2023;33(6):1272–1292. https://doi.org/10.1080/10511482.2021.2020866
9. Berg T, Fuster A, Puri M. Fintech lending. *Annu Rev Financ Econ.* 2022;14(1):187–207. https://doi.org/10.1146/annurev-financial-101521-112042
10. Schwartz AF. *Housing Policy in the United States.* New York, NY: Routledge; 2021. https://doi.org/10.4324/9781003097501
11. Greenberg M. Seeking shelter: how housing and urban exclusion shape exurban disaster. *Sociologica.* 2021;15(1):67–89. https://doi.org/10.6092/issn.1971-8853/11869
12. Greenberg M, Angelo H, Losada E, Wilmers CC. Relational geographies of urban unsustainability: the entanglement of California's housing crisis with WUI growth and climate change. *Proc Natl Acad Sci U S A.* 2024;121(32):e2310080121. https://doi.org/10.1073/pnas.2310080121
13. Casey LS, Reisner SL, Findling MG, et al. Discrimination in the United States: experiences of lesbian, gay, bisexual, transgender, and queer Americans. *Health Serv Res.* 2019;54(suppl 2):1454–1466. https://doi.org/10.1111/1475-6773.13229
14. Fraser B, Pierse N, Chisholm E, Cook H. LGBTIQ+ homelessness: a review of the literature. *Int J Environ Res Public Health.* 2019;16(15):2677. https://doi.org/10.3390/ijerph16152677
15. Committee on Lesbian, Gay, Bisexual, and Transgender Health Issues and Research Gaps and Opportunities; Board on the Health of Select Populations; Institute of Medicine. *The Health of Lesbian, Gay, Bisexual, and Transgender People: Building a Foundation for Better Understanding.* Washington, DC: National Academies Press; 2011.
16. Rice JL, Long J, Levenda A. Against climate apartheid: confronting the persistent legacies of expendability for climate justice. *Environ Plan E Nat Space.* 2022;5(2):625–645. https://doi.org/10.1177/2514848621999286
17. Goldsmith L, Raditz V, Méndez M. Queer and present danger: understanding the disparate impacts of disasters on LGBTQ+ communities. *Disasters.* 2022;46(4):946–973. https://doi.org/10.1111/disa.12509
18. Mann S, McKay T, Gonzales G. Climate change-related disasters & the health of LGBTQ+ populations. *J Clim Change Health.* 2024;18:100304. https://doi.org/10.1016/j.joclim.2024.100304
19. California Health Interview Survey. *CHIS 2023 Methodology Series: Report 2–Data Collection Methods.* Los Angeles, CA: UCLA Center for Health Policy Research; 2024.
20. Schotanus-Dijkstra M, Pieterse ME, Drossaert CHC, et al. What factors are associated with flourishing? Results from a large representative national sample. *J Happiness Stud.* 2016;17(4):1351–1370. https://doi.org/10.1007/s10902-015-9647-3
21. Van Lente E, Barry MM, Molcho M, et al. Measuring population mental health and social well-being. *Int J Public Health.* 2012;57(2):421–430. https://doi.org/10.1007/s00038-011-0317-x
22. California Health Interview Survey. *CHIS 2023 Methodology Series: Report 5–Weighting and Variance Estimation.* Los Angeles, CA: UCLA Center for Health Policy Research; 2024.
23. White BP, Breakey S, Brown MJ, et al. Mental health impacts of climate change among vulnerable populations globally: an integrative review. *Ann Glob Health.* 2023;89(1):66. https://doi.org/10.5334/aogh.4105
24. Lerner RM, Wang J, Hershberg RM, et al. Positive youth development among minority youth: a relational developmental systems model. In: Cabrera NJ, Leyendecker B, eds. *Handbook on Positive Development of Minority Children and Youth.* Cham, Switzerland: Springer; 2017:5–17. https://doi.org/10.1007/978-3-319-43645-6_1
25. Benevolenza MA, DeRigne L. The impact of climate change and natural disasters on vulnerable populations: a systematic review of literature. *J Hum Behav Soc Environ.* 2019;29(2):266–281. https://doi.org/10.1080/10911359.2018.1527739
26. Dundon LA, Camp JS. Climate justice and home-buyout programs: renters as a forgotten population in managed retreat actions. *J Environ Stud Sci.* 2021;11(3):420–433. https://doi.org/10.1007/s13412-021-00691-4
27. Ge S, Johnson S, Tzur-Ilan N. Climate risk, insurance premiums and the effects on mortgage and credit outcomes. Federal Reserve Bank of Dallas. January 2025. Available at: https://www.dallasfed.org/~/media/documents/research/papers/2025/wp2505.pdf. Accessed April 3, 2025.
28. Sastry P, Sen I, Tenekedjieva A-M. When insurers exit: climate losses, fragile insurers, and mortgage markets. Published online December 23, 2023. *SSRN.* https://doi.org/10.2139/ssrn.4674279
29. Monto MA, Neuweiler S. The rise of bisexuality: US representative data show an increase over time in bisexual identity and persons reporting sex with both women and men. *J Sex Res.* 2024;61(6):974–987. https://doi.org/10.1080/00224499.2023.2225176
30. Schulman JK, Erickson-Schroth L. Mental health in sexual minority and transgender women. *Psychiatr Clin North Am.* 2017;40(2):309–319. https://doi.org/10.1016/j.psc.2017.01.011
31. Mahowald L, Shaw A. *Climate Change Risk for LGBT People in the United States.* The Williams Institute, UCLA Schol of Law, 2024. Available at: https://escholarship.org/uc/item/7xw635f3. Accessed April 2, 2025.
32. Pollitt AM, Roberts TS. Internalized binegativity, LGBQ+ community involvement, and definitions of bisexuality. *J Bisex.* 2021;21(3):357–379. https://doi.org/10.1080/15299716.2021.1984363
33. Bosson JK, Vandello JA, Burnaford RM, Weaver JR, Wasti SA. Precarious manhood and displays of physical aggression. *Pers Soc Psychol Bull.* 2009;35(5):623–634. https://doi.org/10.1177/0146167208331161
34. Skidmore WC, Linsenmeier JAW, Bailey JM. Gender nonconformity and psychological distress in lesbians and gay men. *Arch Sex Behav.* 2006;35(6):685–697. https://doi.org/10.1007/s10508-006-9108-5
35. American Civil Liberties Union. *Mapping Attacks on LGBTQ Rights in US State Legislatures in 2025.* Available at: https://www.aclu.org/legislative-attacks-on-lgbtq-rights-2025. Accessed April 3, 2025.

Impact of the January 2025 Los Angeles Firestorm on People Experiencing Homelessness

Evan Michael Shannon, MD, MPH, Jessie Chien, PhD, Danielle Paulazzo, MPH, Gabrielle Arreglo, Benjamin F. Henwood, PhD, MSW, and Randall Kuhn, PhD

See also Climate Change/Natural Disasters, pp. 761–813.

Objectives. To provide a descriptive assessment of self-reported injury and life disruption attributable to the January 2025 Los Angeles County (LAC), California, firestorm among a sample of people experiencing homelessness (PEH).

Methods. We integrated firestorm impact measures into an ongoing longitudinal survey of PEH in LAC. Adult PEH who completed the December 2024 and January 2025 surveys were included.

Results. Among 374 respondents (average age 40 years, 45.7% female, 35.8% Hispanic, 23.5% non-Hispanic Black, 30.2% non-Hispanic White, 84.1% chronically homeless), 286 (76.5%) reported life disruption or injury from the firestorm. Compared with sheltered or housed respondents (n = 144), unsheltered vehicular respondents (n = 111) and unsheltered public respondents (n = 119) were more likely to report having their lives in danger, being injured, damage to living space, having to evacuate, damage or loss of belongings, and difficulty finding shelter. Those in evacuation zones (n = 48) more frequently reported having to evacuate, prolonged smoke exposure, and difficulty finding shelter.

Conclusions. The firestorm caused injury or disruption for most survey participants, especially unsheltered PEH.

Public Health Implications. Wildfire disaster preparedness and response should integrate homeless service coordination, with attention to unsheltered PEH. (*Am J Public Health*. 2026;116(6):790–797. https://doi.org/10.2105/AJPH.2026.308510)

AJPH June 2026, Vol. 116, No. 6

The January 2025 Los Angeles County (LAC), California, wildfires and coinciding extreme wind event (hereafter "firestorm") were among the most devastating urban wildfires in history, destroying an estimated 18 000 structures, displacing 200 000 residents, causing an estimated $275 billion in damages, and leading to 29 deaths.[1] While most coordinated federal, state, and local response efforts focused on mitigating damage sustained by homeowners in affected neighborhoods, people experiencing homelessness (PEH) remained acutely vulnerable. LAC is home to the largest unsheltered population in the United States, with more than 52 000 people living on the streets, in tents or makeshift shelters, or in vehicles on any given night.[2] Despite growing research demonstrating that PEH are at greater risk from the harmful health effects of chronic climate hazards (e.g., extreme heat, air pollution) compared with those with stable housing,[3–6] less is known about how PEH experience acute climate-related natural disasters, such as wildfires.[7]

In the wake of the firestorm, coordination between LAC homelessness services and emergency response systems enabled the evacuation of more than 500 PEH from shelters located in fire danger zones.[8] However, little is known about the firestorm's impact on the county's broader unsheltered population. The objective of this study was to provide a descriptive assessment of injury and life disruption from the January 2025 LAC firestorm among a sample of PEH, using a unique monthly longitudinal survey of LAC's unhoused population that was ongoing when this disaster occurred. We also report differences in firestorm impact by sheltered status and proximity to fire evacuation zones.

METHODS

We analyzed data from the Periodic Assessment of Trajectories of Housing, Homelessness, and Health Study (PATHS), a monthly longitudinal survey of PEH in LAC.[9,10] Launched in December 2021, respondents are primarily recruited annually during the fieldwork for the LAC Homeless Count Demographic Survey, which uses a probability-based sampling design to survey around 4000 unsheltered adults across about 25% of county census tracts and produce representative estimates of LAC's unsheltered population.[11] Upon completion of the survey, respondents are invited to enroll in PATHS, with recruitment supplemented by targeted street outreach at unsheltered hotspots in the 2 months following the survey and, beginning in August 2024, through health care providers serving PEH. Those who express interest are sent a link to a secure website with study information, consent procedures, and a self-administered screening survey. Eligibility criteria include (1) having spent at least 1 night in the past month in a homeless shelter or unsheltered setting (e.g., street, vehicle, tent, or makeshift shelter), (2) residing in LAC, and (3) being aged at least 18 years. Compared with the county's unsheltered population as estimated by the survey, PATHS enrollees as of December 2024 (n = 563) were younger, included a higher proportion of women and non-Hispanic White individuals, and had a lower prevalence of substance use history (Table 1).

Study enrollees receive a text or e-mail every month with a link to a short monthly survey conducted on a secure website accessible by phone or computer and available in English or Spanish. As part of a trauma-informed design, all survey items include a "prefer not to answer" option, with such responses treated as "missing" in analyses.

Exposure

Surveys collect data on shelter status (i.e., unsheltered in public, unsheltered and living in a car, and sheltered or residing in transitional or permanent supportive housing) and current location, which can be provided as addresses, geographic coordinates, or neighborhood of residence (selected from a list of 272 neighborhoods in LAC); addresses and coordinates are subsequently mapped to the list of neighborhoods. Shelter status and proximity to the evacuation order zone were defined using shelter and neighborhood location information reported in the December 2024 monthly survey to

TABLE 1— **Sociodemographic and Self-Reported Clinical Conditions Among the Analytic Sample, Active PATHS Enrollees, and Respondents of the Demographic Survey for the Greater Los Angeles Homeless Count: 2022–2024**

	Mean ±SD or No. (%)		
Characteristic	Survey Participants (n = 374)	Active PATHS Enrollees (n = 563)	Homeless Count (2022–2024; n = 16 253)
Age, y	40 ±11.5	41 ±12.3	44 ±13.2
Race/ethnicity			
Non-Hispanic White	113 (30.2)	162 (28.8)	3847 (23.7)
Non-Hispanic Black/African American	88 (23.5)	129 (22.9)	4605 (28.3)
Any Hispanic/Latino	134 (35.8)	208 (36.9)	6664 (41.0)
Other or multiracial	24 (6.4)	40 (7.1)	1030 (6.3)
Sex			
Male	197 (52.7)	281 (49.9)	11 269 (69.3)
Female	167 (44.7)	267 (47.4)	4497 (27.7)
Other	7 (1.9)	10 (1.8)	488 (3.0)
Substance use history	95 (25.4)	151 (26.8)	5147 (31.7)
Chronically homeless	311 (83.2)	451 (80.1)	12 894 (79.3)

Note. PATHS = Periodic Assessment of Trajectories of Housing, Homelessness, and Health Study. The sample size was n = 374. The sample was derived from PATHS respondents who completed the December 2024 and January 2025 surveys and provided responses to the firestorm and housing status questions. Participants who selected "Prefer not to answer" are not shown in the table but are factored into the column percentages.

approximate participants' circumstances at the time of the January 2025 firestorm, which may have subsequently precipitated changes in shelter status or neighborhood location by the January 2025 survey. Neighborhoods were classified as being in an evacuation order area if at least 10% of their geographic area overlapped with a fire evacuation order zone.

Outcomes

We incorporated a firestorm exposure module into the monthly survey distributed on January 20, 2025 (the wildfire ignited on January 7). Questions in this module were adapted from Harville et al.[12] and included a series of multiple-choice items asking whether the wildfires and extreme winds caused participants to feel that their life was in danger, sustain an injury, experience damage to their living space, evacuate or leave their place of residence, experience more difficulties finding shelter, or suffer damage or loss of their belongings. The module also included a question assessing the extent of respondents' prolonged exposure to wildfire smoke and an optional open-response question inviting respondents to describe the impacts they experienced in their own words. These firestorm questions were administered only in the January 2025 survey wave.

Statistical Analysis

The analytic sample was restricted to participants who completed the December 2024 and January 2025 surveys and reported shelter status in the December survey. We performed descriptive statistics and the χ^2 test to determine associations of shelter status and proximity to fire evacuation order zones with self-reported firestorm impact. In sensitivity analyses, we examined associations using shelter status reported in the January monthly survey; substantive interpretations were similar, so we present results using December shelter status. We completed the analysis in R version 4.4.1 (R Foundation for Statistical Computing, Vienna, Austria); statistical significance was set at $P < .05$, and all tests were 2-tailed. We reviewed and thematically summarized open-ended responses describing firestorm impacts to contextualize the survey findings.

RESULTS

A total of 412 participants completed both December 2024 and January 2025 surveys (459 in December, 440 in January). Data on firestorm exposure and housing status in the previous month were available for 374 (90.8%) respondents, making up our final analytic sample. Of these 374 participants, the mean age was 40 years (SD = 11.5), 167 (44.7%) were female, 134 (35.8%) were Hispanic, 113 (30.2%) were non-Hispanic White, 88 (23.5%) were non-Hispanic Black, and 311 (83.2%) were chronically homeless (i.e., homeless for greater than 1 year; Table 1). Compared with the active PATHS enrollees, the analytic sample was mostly similar across sociodemographic characteristics (Table 1). There were 119 (31.8%) who reported being unsheltered in a public setting (e.g., tents, makeshift shelters, outside) in the previous month, 111 (29.7%) unsheltered and living in a vehicle, and 144 (38.5%) sheltered or housed before the January 2025 firestorm (Table 2).

The geographic distribution of participants as determined by self-reported location (available for 324 [86.6%] respondents) was similar to the distribution of PEH overall based on the LAC Homeless Count Demographic Survey results from 2022–2024 (Table 2).[2] Figure 1 shows the geographic distribution of the analytic sample, along with the perimeters of the January 2025 wildfires (e.g., Eaton, Palisades, and Hurst fires), the areas under evacuation order during that month, and fastest 5-second wind gust for each neighborhood based on the closest National Oceanic and Atmospheric Administration monitoring station. Forty-eight respondents (14.8%) resided in areas that were subject to a fire evacuation order, with higher exposure among sheltered individuals (20.2%) than unsheltered (12.6%; $P = .044$).

Overall, 286 (76.4%) of participants reported any impact from the firestorm; 208 (55.6%) reported their lives were in danger, 172 (46.0%) reported damage to living space, 132 (35.3%) reported walking through smoke for extended periods, 129 (34.5%) reported having to evacuate, 128 (34.2%) reported more difficulty finding shelter, 79 (21.1%) reported being injured, and 43 (11.5%) reported having a friend or family member injured or killed (Figure 2).

Compared with those who were sheltered, unsheltered respondents were more likely to report having their lives in danger (65.5% living in public vs 61.3% living in a vehicle vs 43.1% sheltered; $P < .001$), being injured (31.9% vs 18.9% vs 13.9%; $P = .001$), having damage to living space (75.6% vs 37.8% vs 27.8%; $P < .001$), having to evacuate (48.7% vs 37.8% vs 20.1%; $P < .001$), having damage or loss to belongings (52.9% vs 24.3% vs 15.3%; $P < .001$), or having more difficulty finding shelter compared with those who were sheltered (50.4% vs 33.3% vs 21.5%; $P < .001$; Figure 2). Respondents residing in neighborhoods with areas subject to an evacuation order were more likely to report

TABLE 2— Participant Location by Los Angeles County Service Planning Area (SPA) and Fire Evacuation Zone Status, by Sheltered Status, and With Comparison With Respondents of the Greater Los Angeles Homeless Count Demographic Survey: 2022–2024

	No. (%)				
Characteristic	Overall (n = 374)	Unsheltered-Public (n = 119)	Unsheltered-Vehicle (n = 111)	Sheltered or Housed (n = 144)	Homeless Count (2022–2024; n = 16 253)
Los Angeles County SPA					
Antelope Valley	3 (0.9)	0 (0.0)	1 (1.0)	2 (1.6)	789 (4.9)
San Fernando Valley	68 (21.0)	15 (15.3)	18 (18.6)	35 (27.1)	2173 (13.4)
San Gabriel Valley	20 (6.2)	6 (6.1)	10 (10.3)	4 (3.1)	906 (5.6)
Metro	87 (26.9)	29 (29.6)	18 (18.6)	40 (31.0)	5025 (30.9)
West	47 (14.5)	17 (17.3)	17 (17.5)	13 (10.1)	2491 (15.3)
South	35 (10.8)	15 (15.3)	8 (8.2)	12 (9.3)	2676 (16.5)
East	19 (5.9)	9 (9.2)	6 (6.2)	4 (3.1)	875 (5.4)
South Bay	45 (13.9)	7 (7.1)	19 (19.6)	19 (14.7)	1318 (8.1)
Unknown	50	21	14	15	NA
Fire evacuation status of previous location					
Not in an evacuation order area	276 (85.2)	84 (85.7)	89 (91.8)	103 (79.8)	NA
In an evacuation order area	48 (14.8)	14 (14.3)	8 (8.2)	26 (20.2)	NA
Unknown	50	21	14	15	

Note. NA = not applicable. Shelter status reflects the December monthly survey before the January 2025 firestorm. SPA and fire evacuation status were determined based on neighborhood of residence reported in the December 2024 monthly survey for Periodic Assessment of Trajectories of Housing, Homelessness, and Health Study participants and location where demographic survey was completed for the demographic survey. A neighborhood was considered to be in an evacuation order area if at least 10% of its area overlapped with a fire evacuation order zone. Participants who selected "Prefer not to answer" are not shown in the table but are factored into the column percentages.

having to leave than those residing in neighborhoods without areas under evacuation order (50.0% vs 31.9%; *P* = .015), more likely to report more difficulty finding shelter (47.9% vs 31.9%; *P* = .031), and more likely to experience extended smoke exposure (54.2% vs 34.4%; *P* = .009; Figure 2).

When asked to describe the impacts of the firestorm in their own words, many respondents highlighted the ways the extreme winds and wildfires had compromised their daily routines, access to services, and physical and mental well-being. Consistent with the quantitative findings, unsheltered respondents recounted how falling debris damaged their tents or vehicles and how strong winds swept away their personal belongings. Others reported being forced to leave their sleeping location because of the winds, wildfires, or heavy smoke. Some described being "unable to stay at [their] usual spots" because shelters were damaged or closed under evacuation orders or because many unsheltered locations they frequented were no longer safe.

Respondents also described disruptions to services and continuity of care because of the closure of clinics and other service sites following fire damage or evacuation orders. For example, one participant explained that because their clinic burned down, they were "unable to get prescriptions, change [their] referrals, or speak to [their] provider for updates" (unsheltered Hispanic female, aged 50–60 years). Prolonged exposure to smoke, ash, and toxic air particles emerged as a common concern; many described experiencing breathing difficulties, sore throats, and excessive coughing and wheezing that exacerbated existing conditions like asthma, as well as fear about longer-term health effects from extended smoke exposure. Others expressed fear about future wildfire events; as one respondent wrote: "Sometimes other people around me start fires and I don't know if that's going to spark a big fire like the wildfires we had" (unsheltered Black female, aged 20–30 years).

DISCUSSION

In this study, we found that most respondents reported injury or significant disruption because of the January

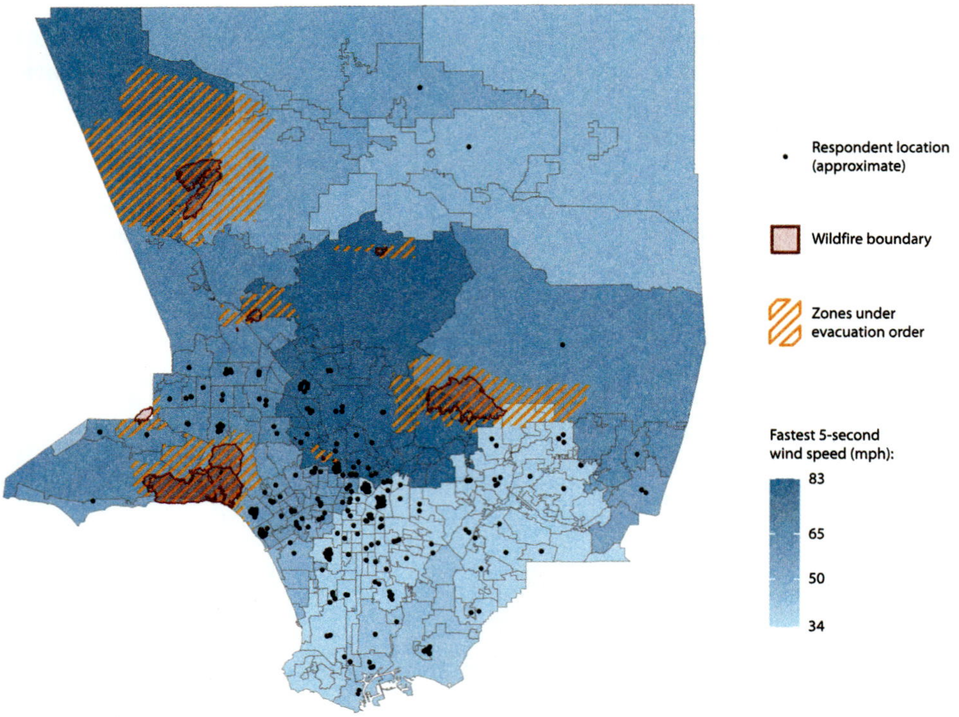

FIGURE 1— Geographic Distribution of Sample Participants Relative to the January 2025 Wildfires, Evacuation Order Areas, and Neighborhood Fastest 5-Second Wind Speed: Los Angeles County

Note. Participant location is based on information reported in the December 2024 monthly survey and was available for 324 participants. Respondent locations are approximate and reflect the centroid of the reported neighborhood of residence. Wildfire and evacuation order zone boundaries reflect the maximum extent observed between January 7 (the first day of the firestorms in Los Angeles County) and January 31, 2025. Wind speed corresponds to the fastest 5-second gust recorded on January 7, 2025, based on data from 14 National Oceanic and Atmospheric Administration monitoring stations across Los Angeles County. Wind measurements were assigned to neighborhoods by calculating neighborhood centroids and linking each centroid to the nearest monitoring station.

2025 firestorm. Unsheltered individuals, especially those living outside, and those residing near evacuation zones reported greater disruptions. However, disruption was widespread across the county, likely reflecting the extreme wind conditions that extended well beyond formal evacuation areas. Quantitative findings were corroborated by qualitative responses, providing a comprehensive account of how the firestorm affected PEH in LAC and offering insights for future wildfire and disaster preparedness.

Although previous literature has documented the unique vulnerability of PEH to climate-related hazards, this study is among the first to empirically examine exposure to urban wildfires. Wildfires differ from other climate hazards in several key ways, including limited predictability and advance warning, prolonged exposure to hazardous conditions, ad hoc evacuation processes, and the extent of damage.[13] These features are particularly salient in the western United States, where wildfires are most common and where unsheltered homelessness is concentrated.[9]

Consistent with conceptual models identifying dwelling type as a moderator of climate-related harm among PEH,[5] unsheltered individuals reported significantly greater disruption than those in shelters. This disparity likely reflects heightened exposure to extreme winds, which participants described as damaging encampments and dispersing personal belongings. Notably, extended smoke exposure did not differ by shelter status, suggesting that wildfire smoke permeated outdoor and indoor environments for PEH, mirroring patterns observed among housed residents in LAC.[14]

This study also contributes novel evidence regarding proximity to evacuation zones, a dimension of exposure specific to wildfires, given their limited geographic footprint relative to hazards such as hurricanes or extreme heat. While only 15% of participants resided within evacuation zones, individuals in these areas reported greater disruption, including more frequent evacuations, prolonged smoke exposure, and increased difficulty accessing shelter.

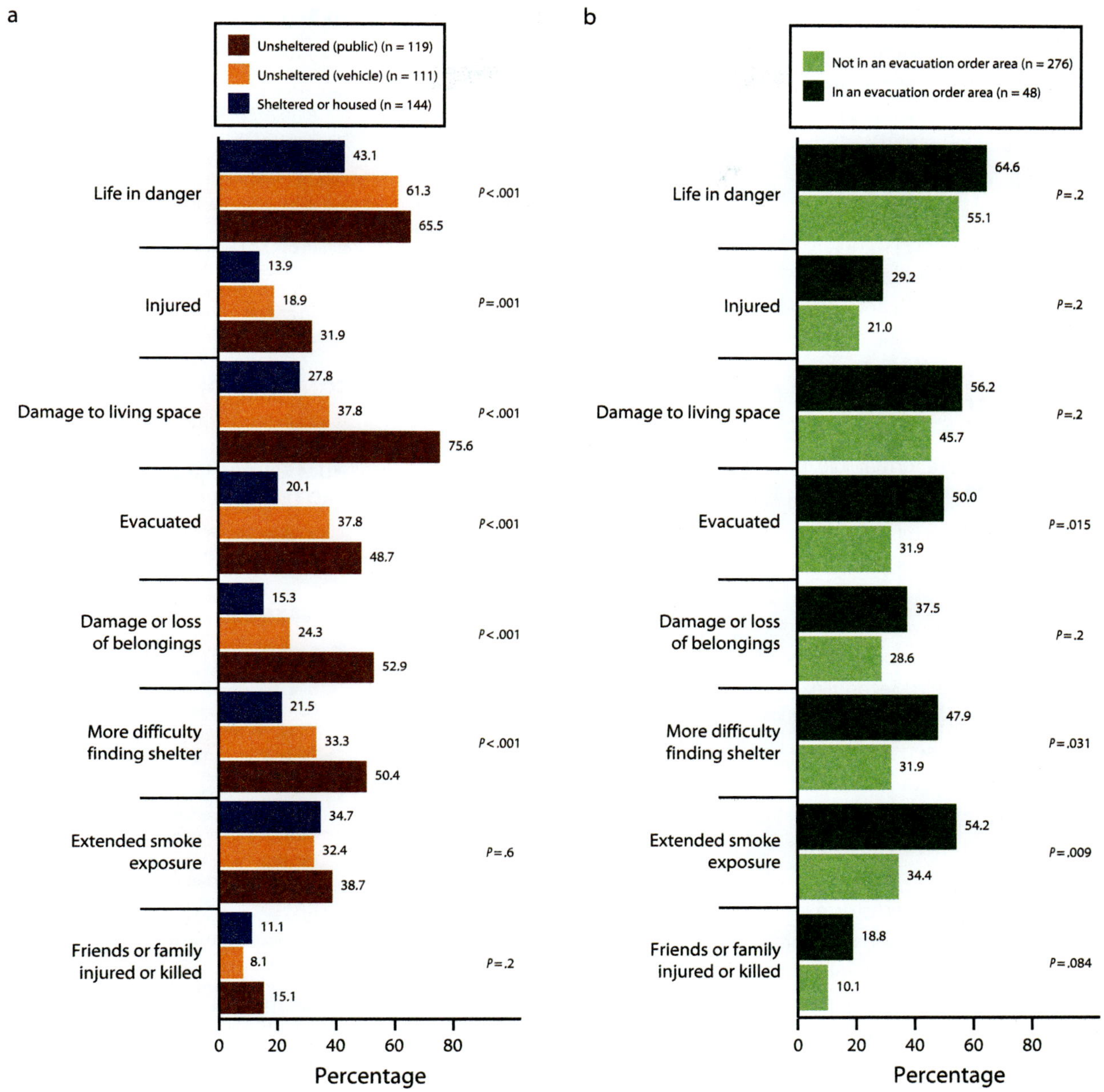

FIGURE 2— **Self-Reported Injury and Life Disruption Among the Analytic Sample, by (a) Shelter Status and (b) Proximity to a Fire Evacuation Order Zone: Los Angeles County, January 2025**

Note. P values are from the χ^2 test. The sample size was n = 374.

Qualitative accounts indicated that shelters and social services near fire-affected areas were closed or damaged, further constraining options. Importantly, high levels of disruption were reported regardless of proximity, underscoring that wildfire impacts extended well beyond formal evacuation boundaries. Future analyses should examine whether underlying vulnerabilities—such as previous displacement or preexisting health conditions—amplified firestorm-related harms.[15]

Although California operates an advanced wildfire response system, this infrastructure does not necessarily target the needs of PEH during urban wildfires. Formally integrating homeless outreach organizations into local emergency operations could reduce disproportionate impacts by facilitating targeted protective measures such as improving emergency shelter availability (especially near evacuation zones), dissemination of protective equipment (e.g., N95s, goggles), and deploying mobile clinics to areas with high concentrations of PEH during wildfires. Furthermore, during the firestorm, mutual aid networks and other self-help organizations played a pivotal role in filling gaps when formal outreach efforts were redirected to establish emergency shelter options, offering the potential for a more formal role in wildfire response.[16]

Several limitations warrant consideration. First, the sample included only PEH with regular smartphone or Internet access, although previous estimates suggest that the majority of PEH have access to a phone.[17] Second, exposure was self-reported rather than derived from remotely sensed meteorological or air quality data. Third, nonresponse bias is possible, particularly if individuals most severely affected were unable to complete surveys. Fourth, the absence of prefirestorm injury data limits comparisons to baseline conditions. Finally, we did not directly assess how disaster coordination functioned with respect to PEH-specific needs.

In conclusion, the convergence of quantitative and qualitative findings indicates substantial impacts of the January 2025 firestorm on PEH, particularly among unsheltered individuals and those living near wildfire activity. These findings highlight the need for more intentional coordination between emergency response systems and homeless service infrastructures to ensure that PEH are adequately protected during future urban wildfires. AJPH

ABOUT THE AUTHORS

Evan Michael Shannon is with the Division of General Internal Medicine and Health Services Research at the David Geffen School of Medicine, University of California, Los Angeles (UCLA). Jessie Chien is with the California Center for Population Research and the Department of Community Health Sciences at the Fielding School of Public Health, UCLA. Danielle Paulazzo was with the Department of Community Health Sciences at the Fielding School of Public Health and the Department of Urban Planning at the Luskin School of Public Affairs, UCLA. Gabrielle Arreglo is with UCLA. Benjamin F. Henwood is with the Suzanne Dworak-Peck School of Social Work, University of Southern California, Los Angeles. Randall Kuhn is with the Department of Community Health Sciences at the Fielding School of Public Health, UCLA.

CORRESPONDENCE

Correspondence should be sent to Evan Michael Shannon, MD, MPH, Division of General Internal Medicine and Health Services Research, 110 Glendon Ave, Suite 850-812, Los Angeles, CA 90024 (e-mail: emshannon@mednet.ucla.edu). Reprints can be ordered at https://www.ajph.org by clicking the "Reprints" link.

PUBLICATION INFORMATION

Full Citation: Shannon EM, Chien J, Paulazzo D, Arreglo G, Henwood BF, Kuhn R. Impact of the January 2025 Los Angeles firestorm on people experiencing homelessness. *Am J Public Health*. 2026;116(6):790–797.

Acceptance Date: February 17, 2026.

DOI: https://doi.org/10.2105/AJPH.2026.308510

ORCID iDs:

Evan Michael Shannon https://orcid.org/0000-0003-0248-7038

Jessie Chien https://orcid.org/0000-0003-4968-2789

Danielle Paulazzo https://orcid.org/0009-0007-0441-965X

Gabrielle Arreglo https://orcid.org/0009-0000-5530-2821

Benjamin F. Henwood https://orcid.org/0000-0001-8346-3569

Randall Kuhn https://orcid.org/0000-0001-5664-6933

CONTRIBUTORS

E. M. Shannon, J. Chien, B. F. Henwood, and R. Kuhn conceptualized and designed the study. D. Paulazzo and G. Arreglo provided invaluable contributions to data acquisition. J. Chien performed the analysis. E. M. Shannon, J. Chien, and R. Kuhn authored the initial drafts of the article. B. F. Henwood provided critical edits to the article for important intellectual content. All authors approved the final version to be published.

ACKNOWLEDGMENTS

The components of the Periodic Assessment of Trajectories of Housing, Homelessness, and Health Study (PATHS) specific to the impact of the firestorm are supported by the National Science Foundation/National Hazards Center Special Call for Health Outcomes and Climate-Related Disaster Research. PATHS is additionally supported by the Hilton Institute and the California Center for Population Research (funded by the National Institute of Child Health and Human Development).

Components of this article were previously presented at the 2025 American Public Health Association Annual Conference in Washington, DC, on November 2, 2025.

CONFLICTS OF INTEREST

The authors declare no conflicts of interest.

HUMAN PARTICIPANT PROTECTION

Study protocols were approved by the UCLA institutional review board.

REFERENCES

1. Casey JA, Gu YM, Schwarz L, et al. The 2025 Los Angeles wildfires and outpatient acute health care utilization. *JAMA Health Forum*. 2025;6(11):e254632. https://doi.org/10.1001/jamahealthforum.2025.4632
2. Los Angeles Homeless Services Authority. 2024 Greater Los Angeles Homeless Count Results. Available at: https://www.lahsa.org/documents?id=8164-2024-greater-los-angeles-homeless-count-results-long-version-.pdf. Accessed March 5, 2025.
3. Bezgrebelna M, McKenzie K, Wells S, et al. Climate change, weather, housing precarity, and homelessness: a systematic review of reviews. *Int J Environ Res Public Health*. 2021;18(11):5812. https://doi.org/10.3390/ijerph18115812
4. Kidd SA, Hajat S, Bezgrebelna M, McKenzie K. The climate change–homelessness nexus. *Lancet*. 2021;397(10286):1693–1694. https://doi.org/10.1016/S0140-6736(21)00834-5
5. Kidd SA, Greco S, McKenzie K. Global climate implications for homelessness: a scoping review. *J Urban Health*. 2021;98(3):385–393. https://doi.org/10.1007/s11524-020-00483-1
6. Ramin B, Svoboda T. Health of the homeless and climate change. *J Urban Health*. 2009;86(4):654–664. https://doi.org/10.1007/s11524-009-9354-7
7. Schwarz L, Nguyen A, Schwarz E, et al. Effects of fine particulate matter from wildfire and non-wildfire sources on emergency-department visits in people who were housed and unhoused in San Diego County (CA, USA) during 2012–20: a time-stratified case–crossover study. *Lancet Planet Health*. 2024;8(11):e906–e914. https://doi.org/10.1016/S2542-5196(24)00239-0
8. Los Angeles County Homeless Services and Housing. The Homeless Initiative's wildfire emergency response. Available at: https://homeless.lacounty.gov/news/the-homeless-initiatives-wildfire-emergency-response. Accessed October 25, 2025.

9. Kuhn R, Henwood B, Chien J. Periodic Assessment of Trajectories of Housing, Homelessness and Health (PATHS): fall 2023 update: encampment sweeps and housing trajectories. UCLA Fielding School of Public Health, USC Suzanne Dworak-Peck School of Social Work. December 12, 2023. Available at: https://escholarship.org/uc/item/46n649n0. Accessed January 12, 2026.
10. Padwa H, Chien J, Henwood BF, Cousins SJ, Zakher E, Kuhn R. Homelessness, discrimination, and violent victimization in Los Angeles County. *Am J Prev Med.* 2024;67(5):666–675. https://doi.org/10.1016/j.amepre.2024.06.016
11. Henwood B, Hickey S, Kwack S, Gonzalez AL, Stein A, Kuhn R. 2024 Los Angeles Continuum of Care Homeless Count: Methodology Report. USC Suzanne Dworak-Peck School of Social Work; 2024. Available at: https://dworakpeck.usc.edu/sites/default/files/2024-07/Final%202024%20USC%20Homeless%20Count%20Methodology%20Report_20240716.pdf. Accessed May 6, 2025.
12. Harville EW, Jacobs M, Boynton-Jarrett R. When is exposure to a natural disaster traumatic? Comparison of a trauma questionnaire and disaster exposure inventory. *PLoS One.* 2015;10(4):e0123632. https://doi.org/10.1371/journal.pone.0123632
13. D'Evelyn SM, Jung J, Alvarado E, et al. Wildfire, smoke exposure, human health, and environmental justice need to be integrated into forest restoration and management. *Curr Environ Health Rep.* 2022;9(3):366–385. https://doi.org/10.1007/s40572-022-00355-7
14. Benmarhnia T, Errett NA, Casey JA. Beneath the smoke: understanding the public health impacts of the Los Angeles urban wildfires. *Environ Epidemiol.* 2025;9(3):e388. https://doi.org/10.1097/EE9.0000000000000388
15. Patanwala MY, Garcia CM, Kushel M. Health care for people experiencing homelessness. *JAMA.* 2024;332(1):70–71. https://doi.org/10.1001/jama.2024.5213
16. Mitchell S. Mutual aid networks that emerged in housing crisis are mobilizing amid LA fires. Truthout. January 16, 2025. Available at: https://truthout.org/articles/mutual-aid-networks-that-emerged-in-housing-crisis-are-mobilizing-amid-la-fires. Accessed October 20, 2025.
17. Rhoades H, Wenzel SL, Rice E, Winetrobe H, Henwood B. No digital divide? Technology use among homeless adults. *J Soc Distress Homeless.* 2017;26(1):73–77. https://doi.org/10.1080/10530789.2017.1305140

Heat-Related Emergency Medical Services Activations in the United States, 2020–2024: Rates, Demographics, and Geographic Distribution

Shubhayu Saha, PhD, Lauren Jensen, MPH, MCRP, Cody S. Olsen, MS, Casey Gregor, Benjamin Fisher, MPA, John Balbus, MD, MPH, Arsenio Mataka, JD, and N. Clay Mann, PhD, MS, MBA

See also Climate Change/Natural Disasters, pp. 761–813.

AJPH June 2026, Vol. 116, No. 6

Objectives. To examine the magnitude of heat-related emergency medical services (EMS) activations across the United States and identify factors that increase the risk of heat exposure illness.

Methods. We extracted heat-related EMS activations from April through September for 2020 through 2024 from the National Emergency Medical Services Information System (NEMSIS) database. We linked information from the 2022 Centers for Disease Control and Prevention (CDC) Social Vulnerability Index with heat-related EMS activations using county of residence. Our analysis focused on heat-related illness by patient demographic, geographic, and EMS system factors.

Results. Among the 79 077 804 EMS activations meeting study inclusion criteria, 261 687 (0.3%) were heat related. The rate of heat-related EMS activations was 16.46 per 100 000 population, with higher rates among older adults, males, African Americans, and Native Hawaiians/Pacific Islanders. Rates were higher in rural counties and in counties characterized by the CDC Social Vulnerability Index as having relatively worse socioeconomic or environmental conditions. Heat-related EMS activations were commonly reported in the afternoon and in indoor locations.

Conclusions. The NEMSIS database provides novel information that improves our ability to monitor heat-related adverse health outcomes.

Public Health Implications. The timely collection and sharing of data provide critical situational awareness to inform public health response efforts during a heat wave. (*Am J Public Health.* 2026;116(6): 798–805. https://doi.org/10.2105/AJPH.2026.308513)

The year 2024 was the hottest on record globally since recordkeeping began in 1850, with average land and ocean surface temperatures 2.32°F (1.29°C) above the 20th-century average.[1] Heat events are increasing in frequency, severity, and duration, and there is growing evidence of the broad-ranging adverse health impacts associated with exposure to extreme heat.[2] There is also broad recognition that deaths and illnesses associated with extreme heat are preventable.[3] Although heat can negatively affect everyone, it does not affect everyone equally. Most of these adverse outcomes are strongly connected to localized factors—housing conditions, neighborhood characteristics, health care access, and social support networks—that amplify the health risks posed by heat exposure.[4]

One important factor that can improve our ability to effectively prepare communities for heat and respond during heat events is the availability of fine-scaled and timely health data related to heat exposure. The US Centers for Disease Control and Prevention (CDC) National Syndromic Surveillance Program captures data on heat-related emergency department (ED) visits.[5] However, the program does not provide data on patients who suffer heat-related illness and are treated by emergency medical services (EMS) professionals but are not transported to an acute care medical facility. In addition, the publicly available heat-related ED data from the program are available only at a coarse spatial scale for the 10 regions defined by the US Department of Health and Human Services. The US Department of Transportation's National Highway Traffic Safety Administration's National Emergency Medical Services Information System (NEMSIS) database is unique in providing nationally consistent and locally resolved information on adverse heat-related illness that requires care provided by local EMS providers in the prehospital setting.

Because these data are available in near real time, they provide a critical, relatively fine-scaled snapshot of surges in health care needs during heat waves to inform short-term responses. In addition, the availability of such data across years allows us to identify specific areas of the country where heat-related illnesses are consistently high and to assess demographic risk factors for those most frequently requiring emergency care because of heat exposure. There are unique elements of the EMS data that help us understand the time and place of EMS response that can inform both short-term and long-term interventions that better protect people suffering from heat exposure.

METHODS

We performed a retrospective analysis of the combined 2020–2024 NEMSIS public research data sets for April to September. NEMSIS is a national database of EMS responses in the United States. NEMSIS collects electronic health record data and standardizes it for research and performance improvement. EMS in all 50 states and the District of Columbia voluntarily collect data at the state level and report them nationally, covering more than 96% of the US population. The data are then de-identified for research purposes. The data contain patient demographic information, response characteristics, location information (including county and zip code of the incident and patient residence), clinical presentations, interventions, and prehospital outcome data. Further details regarding NEMSIS are described elsewhere.[6]

Patient Population

We used guidelines produced by the Council for State and Territorial Epidemiologists for identifying patients with heat-related illness.[7] We included patients whom we suspected experienced a heat-related emergency event when initially treated by an EMS clinician. The event may have occurred indoors or outdoors. We included EMS activations documented by EMS clinicians as having a symptom, cause of injury, or impression with an *ICD-10-CM* (National Center for Health Statistics. *International Classification of Diseases, Tenth Revision, Clinical Modification.* Centers for Disease Control and Prevention. Updated 2024. https://www.cdc.gov/nchs/icd/icd-10-cm/?CDC_AAref_Val) code in the T67 (heatstroke, cramp, exhaustion, etc.), X30 (exposure to excessive natural heat), X32 (exposure to sunlight), or L55 (sunburn) series.

In addition, we included EMS activations with documented use of treatment protocols for heat exposure or exhaustion or for heatstroke or hyperthermia.[8] We also limited EMS activations to states and incident counties consistently submitting data to NEMSIS for a given year. Because the NEMSIS data set may include multiple resource activations for the same patient (e.g., first responder and ambulance transport), we further limited EMS activations to the initial responder (definition in Table A, available as a supplement to the online version of this article at http://www.ajph.org). We identified a comparison group of non–heat-related EMS events with identical inclusion criteria but lacking heat relatedness.

Variables

We analyzed patient characteristics recorded in the EMS record, including sex, race/ethnicity, age, activation time (categorized as 00:00–05:59, 06:00–11:59, 12:00–17:59, or 18:00–23:59), initial patient acuity, patient transported (yes vs no), type of destination, hospital inpatient destination, and hospital capability), and location (using *ICD-10-CM* codes for location of response; Table A). We assigned urbanicity by linking the incident county with Urban Influence Codes.[9] We linked NEMSIS data to Social Vulnerability Index (SVI) data[10] at the county level using residence county if available and incident county otherwise. We categorized the SVI data into quartiles for analysis, with the first quartile being the least vulnerable and the fourth quartile being the most vulnerable counties.

We calculated rates of heat-related EMS activations and all EMS activations per 100 000 population using estimates from the American Community Survey (2022, 5-year estimates, obtained from Integrated Public Use Microdata Series, National Historical Geographic

Information System, University of Minnesota).[11] We calculated yearly population estimates to limit calculations to states submitting to NEMSIS and to zip codes with EMS responses within a given year. This way, yearly rates of EMS activations had denominators that matched numerators geographically. We combined race categories, which are collected as multiselect in NEMSIS and include Hispanic or Latino ethnicity as an option, to match the American Community Survey race categories for reporting as population rates without a Hispanic or Latino category. When multiple race categories were selected, we categorized the EMS activation as 2 or more races.

Statistical Analyses

We estimated rates of all EMS activations along with rates of heat-related EMS activations per 100 000 population overall and by age groups (0–14, 15–64, and 65 years and older). We also estimated rates by sex, race, urbanicity, and SVI quartile. We compared the distributions of patient characteristics (initial acuity, transported, activation time, and location) of heat-related EMS activations with those of non–heat-related EMS activations using bar charts. We tested differences using the χ^2 test.

We calculated average yearly rates of heat-related EMS activations by county by rolling up zip code–level estimates. We included counties if they had at least 1 year of NEMSIS data with a rate of 1 or more heat-related EMS activations per 100 000 population. We excluded years with less than 1 per 100 000 population from county yearly averages, resulting in some very rural counties being excluded. We excluded data from 2020 through 2021 from this rate analysis because 4 states (DE, HI, ID, MA) did not submit data in those years. We mapped counties based on the average yearly rates of heat-related EMS activations categorized into quintiles. We performed analyses using SAS/STAT version 9.4 (SAS Institute Inc, Cary, NC) and R version 4.3.2 (RStudio, Boston, MA). We used a significance level of .001 to determine statistical significance.

RESULTS

We compared descriptive statistics for heat-related EMS activations with all EMS activations for the demographic, geographic, and SVI indicators (Table 1). During the study period, there were 79 077 804 EMS activations that met the study inclusion criteria of a 911-initiated emergency response. Of these activations, 261 687 (0.3%) were heat related, with an annual average rate of 16.46 activations per 100 000 population. Over the course of the study, we identified 32 854 heat-related EMS activations in 2020, 37 274 in 2021, 46 395 in 2022, 70 300 in 2023, and 74 864 in 2024.

Total percentages of heat activations among patients aged 0 to 14 years, 15 to 64 years, and 65 years and older were 5%, 66%, and 28%, respectively; however, the rate of heat activations was highest among those aged 65 years or older (28.03 per 100 000), followed by 15 to 64 years (16.75 per 100 000) and 0 to 14 years (4.66 per 100 000). Rates were higher among males (21.00) than females (11.77), which differs from the pattern observed for all EMS activations. Like all EMS activations, rates of heat-related activations were higher among the Black or African American (23.92) and the Native Hawaiian and other Pacific Islander (23.85) groups. Rates of heat activations were highest in rural counties (21.76) and lowest in urban counties (15.26), as was observed for all EMS activations. Rates of heat activations were highest among patients living in counties that were ranked most vulnerable by the SVI in the fourth quartile (18.22) compared with the first quartile (15.27).

Clinical and EMS system characteristics for heat-related EMS activations differed from those for non–heat-related EMS activations (the Pearson χ^2 test for overall distributional differences across initial acuity, transport, location, and activation time was $P \le .001$ for all; Figure 1). In terms of observed proportions, heat-related EMS activations had a higher proportion classified as emergent or critical than did non–heat-related EMS activations (emergent: 25% heat vs 16% nonheat; critical: 3.9% heat vs 2.8% nonheat). Patients in heat-related EMS activations were transported to a medical facility at nearly the same frequency as those in non–heat-related EMS activations (69.6% heat; 69.1% nonheat). Based on the incident location (described in Table B, available as a supplement to the online version of this article at http://www.ajph.org), heat-related EMS activations were considered outdoors (29%) and occupational (18%) more often than non–heat-related EMS activations (12% outdoors; 10% occupational). However, like non–heat-related EMS activations, indoors was the most common location of response (47% of heat related; 74% of non–heat related). Sports locations made up 3.9% of heat-related EMS activation response locations compared with 0.3% of non–heat-related activations.

The map in Figure 2 displays counties reporting the highest rates of heat activations during the most recent 3 years in the study period. These counties have a wide geographic distribution, including many counties in the northern

TABLE 1— Rates of All and Heat-Related EMS Activations by Demographic, Geographic, and SVI Characteristics: United States, 2020–2024

Characteristic[a]	Rate of All EMS Activations per 100 000 Population (n = 79 077 804)	Rate of Heat-Related EMS Activations per 100 000 Population			
		All Heat-Related (n = 261 687)	Aged 0–14 y (n = 13 535)	Aged 15–64 y (n = 173 644)	Aged 65 y and older (n = 73 722)
National rate	4 974.03	16.46	4.66	16.75	28.03
Sex					
Female	4 696.44	11.77	4.64	11.20	20.71
Male	4 557.70	21.00	4.64	22.08	36.86
Race					
American Indian/Alaska Native	4 256.79	16.50	5.95	18.29	26.28
Asian	1 061.47	3.14	1.69	2.75	7.05
Black/African American	6 873.16	23.92	7.37	25.13	44.44
Native Hawaiian/Other Pacific Islander	6 320.99	23.85	9.55	23.43	57.81
White	3 598.19	13.29	3.39	13.03	22.24
≥ 2 races	169.53	0.43	0.25	0.45	0.92
Urbanicity					
Urban	4 506.50	15.26	4.41	15.57	26.41
Suburban	5 013.56	19.52	5.40	20.21	30.24
Rural	4 978.41	21.76	5.55	22.61	33.81
Frontier	4 875.65	21.38	5.77	21.31	33.57
SVI: Overall, quartile					
1st	3 964.34	15.27	5.63	14.21	28.94
2nd	4 148.14	13.76	4.17	13.62	24.26
3rd	4 860.28	16.21	4.18	16.57	27.26
4th	4 992.00	18.22	4.79	19.43	30.03

Note. ACS = American Community Survey; EMS = emergency medical services; SVI = Social Vulnerability Index; NEMSIS = National Emergency Medical Services Information System. Data include EMS activations reported to NEMSIS during April–September 2020–2024, limited to emergency responses with patient contact in which the reporting EMS unit was first on scene. We identified heat-related activations by documentation of heat-related symptoms (primary or secondary), provider impression, or cause of injury. We calculated rates using ACS 2022 5-year population estimates restricted to zip codes with eligible EMS activations, representing an average annual population of 318 million (96% of the US population of 331 million). Data were available from Washington, DC, and 46 states in 2020–2021, 48 states in 2022, and all 50 states in 2023–2024, representing 92% of the US population in 2020 and 99.7% in 2024. We excluded activations with unknown values for sex, age, race, urbanicity, or SVI from rate calculations.
[a]Characteristics are unknown in NEMSIS for age 6.2%, sex 6.4%, race 31.3% (of whom 24.6% were Hispanic/Latino), urbanicity 2.0%, and SVI 1.1%. Among heat-related EMS activations, NEMSIS characteristics are unknown for age 0.3%, sex 0.5%, race 25.7% (of whom 36.6% were Hispanic/Latino), urbanicity 2.3%, and SVI 1.3%.

regions of the country, indicating that health risks from exposure to heat are observed not just in places where heat is common but also in places that are less accustomed to high temperatures during the summer months.

DISCUSSION

The monitoring of heat-related EMS activations provides novel national surveillance information on the geographic distribution and temporal trends of health impacts from extreme heat. This analysis corroborates existing knowledge of the impact of heat among sociodemographic groups and adds to our understanding of the time, location, and severity of heat-related EMS calls, which can inform local heat preparedness and response efforts. The average annual rates of heat-related EMS activations are similar to estimates of national rates of heat-related ED visits using 2006 through 2010 data.[12] The analysis aligns with our existing understanding that rates of heat-related deaths[13] and ED visits[14] are more common among males. Although the number of heat-related EMS activations was highest in the working age group (15–64 years), which aligns with previous research,[15] the

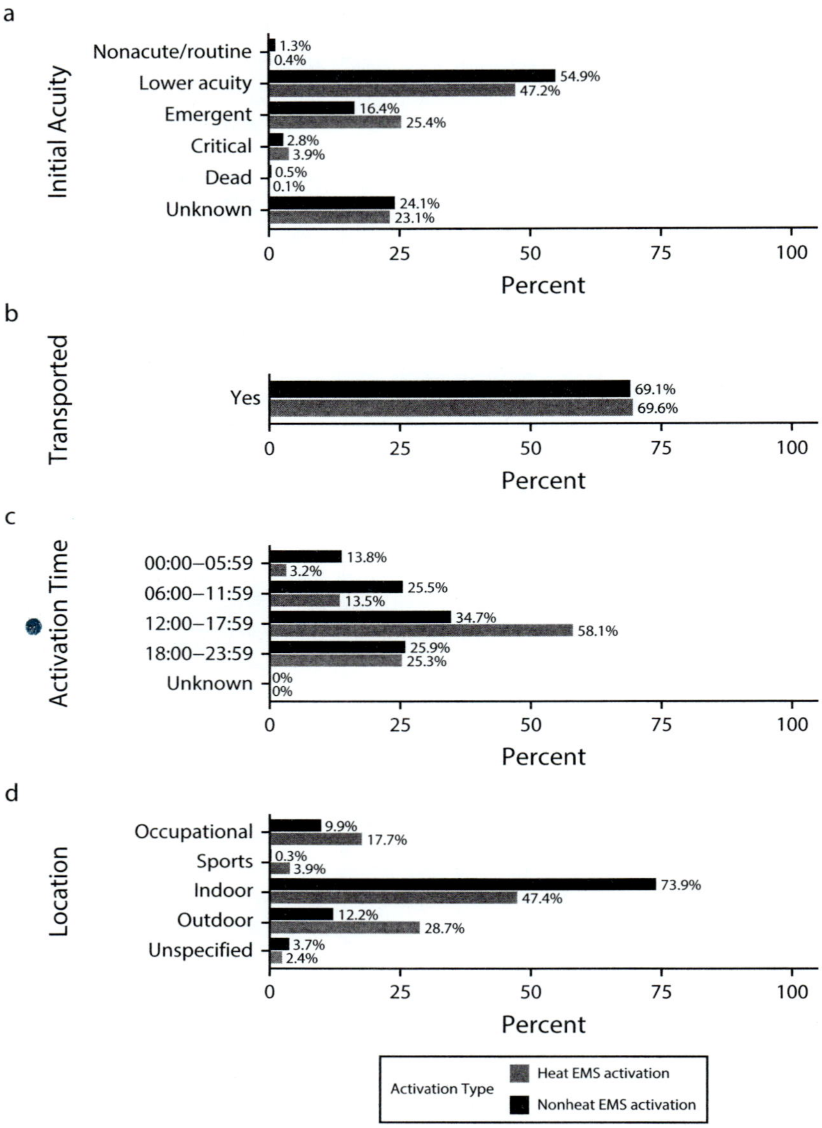

FIGURE 1— Heat-Related Compared With Non–Heat-Related EMS Activations by (a) Initial Acuity, (b) Transported to a Medical Facility, (c) Activation Time, and (d) Location: United States, 2020–2024

Note. EMS = emergency medical services.

rate of heat-related EMS activations was highest in the group aged 65 years and older, which differs from the pattern observed in national heat-related ED visits.

Additionally, the rates were higher in rural than urban counties, which is also supported by current literature evaluating heat-related ED visits.[16] Previous research found more acute outcomes among heat-related EMS activations in rural areas.[17] Lastly, we found that heat-related EMS activations were more often emergent or critical compared with non–heat-related EMS activations, demonstrating the need for additional training and resources for EMS personnel to be able to effectively and promptly treat patients experiencing heat-related illness. Similarly, a study of heat-related EMS activations in Austin-Travis County, Texas, found the need for increased resources and staffing during periods of high temperatures to protect public health.[18] Innovative trends in protocols that encourage the cooling of these critical heat patients before transport, versus immediate and rapid transport as has traditionally been the case, are intended "to reduce the end-organ

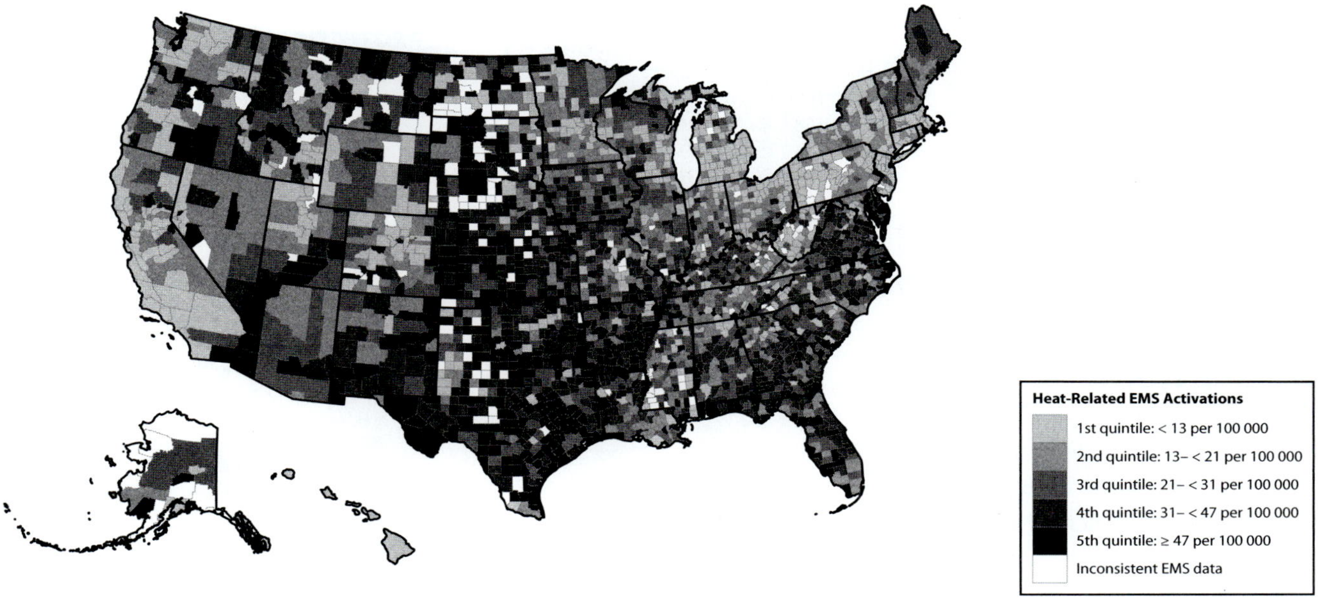

FIGURE 2— Average Yearly Rates of Heat-Related EMS Activations per 100 000 Population: United States, 2020–2024

Note. EMS = emergency medical services.

dysfunction, morbidity, and mortality of severe hyperthermia."[19] The longer scene times have the potential to result in delays in EMS units responding to other requests for EMS if there is not a sufficient number of available units, highlighting the potential need for additional resources during predicted heat waves.

The utility of using the NEMSIS database to inform public policy has been demonstrated through the recent publication of 2 federal geospatial tools. The National Heat-Related EMS Activation Surveillance Dashboard, published in August 2023, provides novel county-level information over the last 2 and 4 weeks on heat-related EMS activations to state and local public health officials and other decision-makers for timely and targeted outreach and assistance.[20] Since the launch of the National Heat-Related EMS Activation Surveillance Dashboard in August 2023, there have been more than 30 000 visits to the dashboard through the end of 2024. Although this tool is able to provide only national-level demographic data, such as age and race of patients through the National Disparity Explorer, the heat-related EMS data and additional demographic data are also integrated into the Heat and Health Index launched in May 2024 by the US Department of Health and Human Services and the CDC.[21] The Heat and Health Index combines aggregated heat-related EMS activations from 2021 through 2023 at the zip code level with data on community characteristics, preexisting health conditions, sociodemographic information, and characteristics of the natural and built environment to provide a national ranking of zip codes. The Heat and Health Index is useful for identifying areas of the country where localized investments in heat risk reduction strategies could protect public health.

There are some limitations associated with using the NEMSIS database that are worth mentioning. The heat-related activations in the NEMSIS database are based on the clinical judgment of EMS providers; however, providers are not required to document the ambient temperature associated with the event. Additionally, we used 911 EMS responses, so we did not include heat-related events without involvement of 911 emergency services in our sample. NEMSIS currently represents all 50 states; however, different states began submitting to NEMSIS at various times, and only 46 states submitted data across the entire study period. For the years 2020 through 2021, the states Delaware, Hawaii, Idaho, and Massachusetts did not report EMS data; thus, we did not include these associated populations in rate analyses for these years. Furthermore, heat illness and injury rates are based on resident populations; thus, geographic burdens of heat-related EMS activations may be overestimated in areas with visiting populations (e.g., amusement parks, festivals). Clinicians often collect EMS

AJPH June 2026, Vol. 116, No. 6

data during patient emergencies; the data are therefore subject to error and nonrandom missingness. Finally, the NEMSIS data rarely include hospital outcomes for transported patients, so we were unable to accurately assess the lethality of heat-related EMS activations.

PUBLIC HEALTH IMPLICATIONS

EMS data for the past 5 years show that high rates of heat-related EMS activations have been observed across the country, indicating that individuals and their communities are unprepared to cope during heat waves, irrespective of whether high temperatures are a common phenomenon where they live. Routine documentation and sharing of heat-related EMS activations provide timely information to improve short-term response efforts during heat waves and to better prepare for surges in health care utilization. Monitoring trends in heat-related adverse outcomes will also guide the implementation of targeted local interventions that can minimize risk factors and reduce heat-related illness and death. AJPH

ABOUT THE AUTHORS

Shubhayu Saha is with Tracking California, Public Health Institute, Oakland, CA. John Balbus is Principal at Climate Care Consulting, Washington DC. During the formative part of the article, Lauren Jensen and Arsenio Mataka were with the US Department of Health and Human Services, Washington, DC. Cody S. Olsen, Casey Gregor, and Benjamin Fisher are with the Utah Data Coordinating Center, University of Utah, Salt Lake City. N. Clay Mann is with the Department of Pediatrics, University of Utah School of Medicine, Salt Lake City.

CORRESPONDENCE

Correspondence should be sent to N. Clay Mann, PhD, MS, MBA, Department of Pediatrics, University of Utah School of Medicine, 295 Chipeta Way, PO Box 581289, Salt Lake City, UT 84158 (e-mail: clay.mann@hsc.utah.edu).

PUBLICATION INFORMATION

Full Citation: Saha S, Jensen L, Olsen CS, et al. Heat-related emergency medical services activations in the United States, 2020–2024: rates, demographics, and geographic distribution. *Am J Public Health*. 2026;116(6):798–805.

Acceptance Date: February 18, 2026.

DOI: https://doi.org/10.2105/AJPH.2026.308513

ORCID iDs:

Shubhayu Saha https://orcid.org/0000-0002-4770-8773

Lauren Jensen https://orcid.org/0000-0002-9525-6214

Cody S. Olsen https://orcid.org/0000-0003-2994-7946

Casey Gregor https://orcid.org/0009-0001-4790-5259

Benjamin Fisher https://orcid.org/0000-0001-6966-5201

John Balbus https://orcid.org/0000-0003-3356-8332

N. Clay Mann https://orcid.org/0000-0003-0727-1965

CONTRIBUTORS

S. Saha, C. S. Olsen, and N. C. Mann conceptualized and designed the study, led the data collection and analysis, and drafted the initial article. S. Saha and N. C. Mann provided project oversight and administration, secured funding, and provided critical feedback throughout the writing process. L. Jensen, J. Balbus, and A. Mataka assisted with the study design, provided data interpretation, and provided the initial review and editing of the article for intellectual content. C. S. Olsen, C. Gregor, and B. Fisher provided technical expertise, supported data visualization and statistical modeling, and contributed to additional article revisions. All authors read and approved the final version of the article and agree to be accountable for all aspects of the work.

ACKNOWLEDGMENTS

We acknowledge and thank all the participating emergency medical services (EMS) clinicians, EMS agencies, and state EMS offices that supported and provided data to the National Emergency Medical Services Information System database.

Note. The authors alone are responsible for the contents and writing of this article. The content has not been cleared by the Department of Health and Human Services and does not necessarily represent the official position of the agency.

CONFLICTS OF INTEREST

The authors have no conflicts of interest to report.

HUMAN PARTICIPANT PROTECTION

The University of Utah institutional review board deemed this study exempt from human participant review because we used de-identified data.

REFERENCES

1. National Oceanic and Atmospheric Administration. 2024 was the world's warmest year on record. January 10, 2025. Available at: https://www.noaa.gov/news/2024-was-worlds-warmest-year-on-record#:~:text=It's%20official%3A%202024%20was%20the,extent%20(coverage)%20on%20record. Accessed May 28, 2025.
2. Ebi KL, Capon A, Berry P, et al. Hot weather and heat extremes: health risks. *Lancet*. 2021;398(10301):698–708. https://doi.org/10.1016/S0140-6736(21)01208-3
3. Centers for Disease Control and Prevention. Temperature extremes. March 2, 2024. Available at: https://www.cdc.gov/climate-health/php/effects/temperature-extremes.html. Accessed May 28, 2025.
4. Niu Y, Li Z, Gao Y, et al. A systematic review of the development and validation of the heat vulnerability index: major factors, methods, and spatial units. *Curr Clim Change Rep*. 2021;7(3):87–97. https://doi.org/10.1007/s40641-021-00173-3
5. Centers for Disease Control and Prevention. Exploring tangible health impact from heat. January 12, 2026. Available at: https://www.cdc.gov/nssp/php/partnerships/health-impact-from-heat-waves.html. Accessed March 28, 2026.
6. Ehlers J, Fisher B, Peterson S, et al. Description of the 2020 NEMSIS public-release research data set. *Prehosp Emerg Care*. 2023;27(4):473–481. https://doi.org/10.1080/10903127.2022.2079779
7. Council of State and Territorial Epidemiologists. Heat-related illness syndrome query: a guidance document for implementing heat-related illness syndromic surveillance in public health practice. September 2016. Available at: https://knowledgerepository.syndromicsurveillance.org/sites/default/files/2022-10/SyndromicSurveillance_CSTEGuidanceDocument_HeatRelatedIllness.pdf. Accessed May 28, 2025.
8. Heat-related EMS activation surveillance dashboard (EMS HeatTracker) companion guide. May 5, 2025. Available at: https://wiki.utahdcc.org/confluence/spaces/NTD/pages/206274695/Heat-Related+EMS+Activation+Surveillance+Dashboard+EMS+HeatTracker+Companion+Guide. Accessed May 28, 2025.
9. US Department of Agriculture Economic Research Service. Urban influence codes. January 7, 2025. Available at: https://www.ers.usda.gov/data-products/urban-influence-codes. Accessed May 28, 2025.
10. Agency for Toxic Substances and Disease Registry. Place and health—Geospatial Research, Analysis, and Services Program. 2024. Available at: https://www.atsdr.cdc.gov/place-health/php/svi/svi-data-documentation-download.html?CDC_AAref_Val. Accessed June 24, 2024.
11. Manson S, Schroeder J, Van Riper D, et al. IPUMS National Historical Geographic Information System: Version 19.0. 2024. Available at: https://doi.org/10.18128/D050.V19.0. Accessed March 28, 2026.

12. Hess JJ, Saha S, Luber G. Summertime acute heat illness in US emergency departments from 2006 through 2010: analysis of a nationally representative sample. *Environ Health Perspect.* 2014;122(11): 1209–1215. https://pmc.ncbi.nlm.nih.gov/articles/PMC4216158
13. Centers for Disease Control and Prevention. Heat-related deaths—United States, 2004–2018. *MMWR Morb Mortal Wkly Rep.* 2020;69(24): 729–734. https://doi.org/10.15585/mmwr.mm6924a1
14. Centers for Disease Control and Prevention. Heat-related emergency department visits—United States, May–September 2023. *MMWR Morb Mortal Wkly Rep.* 2024;73(15):324–329. https://doi.org/10.15585/mmwr.mm7315a1
15. Yeargin S, Hirschhorn R, Grundstein A. Heat-related illnesses transported by United States emergency medical services. *Medicina (Kaunas).* 2020;56(10):543. https://doi.org/10.3390/medicina56100543
16. Sun S, Weinberger KR, Nori-Sarma A, et al. Ambient heat and risks of emergency department visits among adults in the United States: time stratified case crossover study. *BMJ.* 2021;375: e065653. https://doi.org/10.1136/bmj-2021-065653
17. Ahn M, Keith L, Brown HE. Rural heat health disparities: evidence from the US National Emergency Medical Services Information System (NEMSIS). *J Clim Chang Health.* 2025;22:100432. https://doi.org/10.1016/j.joclim.2025.100432
18. Seong K, Jiao J, Mandalapu A. Hourly associations between heat index and heat-related emergency medical service (EMS) calls in Austin–Travis County, Texas. *Int J Environ Res Public Health.* 2023; 20(19):6853. https://doi.org/10.3390/ijerph20196853
19. Stevens E. Article bites #41: consensus statement—prehospital care of exertional heat stroke. July 14, 2022. Available at: https://naemsp.org/2022-7-13-article-bites-41-consensus-statement-prehospital-care-of-exertional-heat-stroke. Accessed July 28, 2025.
20. National Emergency Medical Services Information System. Heat-related EMS activation surveillance dashboard. Available at: https://nemsis.org/heat-related-ems-activation-surveillance-dashboard. Accessed May 28, 2025.
21. Centers for Disease Control and Prevention. Heat and health index. Available at: https://ephtracking.cdc.gov/Applications/heatTracker/?page=detail3. Accessed May 28, 2025.

Emergency Department Burden of Mental Health and Substance Misuse After Hurricane Helene: Insights From Rural Appalachia

Margaret M. Sugg, PhD, MA, Sophia C. Ryan, MA, Annie Preaux, PhD, MPH, Christine Quattro, PhD, MS, AM, Ben Alexander-Eitzman, PhD, MSW, Martie P. Thompson, PhD, Adam Hege, PhD, MPA, and Jennifer D. Runkle, PhD, MSPH

See also Climate Change/Natural Disasters, pp. 761–813.

Objectives. To quantify temporal changes in mental health and substance use emergency department utilization following Hurricane Helene (September 2024) in Western North Carolina and identify disparities across vulnerable populations.

Methods. We conducted a cross-sectional analysis using emergency department surveillance data from Western North Carolina counties. We calculated incidence rate ratios (IRRs) with 95% confidence intervals (CIs) by comparing 3 recovery periods (immediate, early, short-term) with their corresponding calendar dates in 2023.

Results. Alcohol-related visits increased across all periods (immediate: IRR = 1.35; 95% CI = 1.14, 1.60; early: IRR = 1.47; 95% CI = 1.31, 1.65; short-term: IRR = 1.36; 95% CI = 1.21, 1.52). Anxiety disorders increased across all periods, mood disorders increased during early recovery, schizophrenia visits increased during short-term recovery (IRR = 1.19; 95% CI = 1.02, 1.40), and opioid-related visits showed marginally significant increases during short-term recovery (IRR = 1.21; 95% CI = 1.00, 1.45). Counties with higher elderly populations showed amplified alcohol and anxiety effects; counties with higher uninsured or covered by Medicaid rates showed lower utilization.

Conclusions. Hurricane Helene was associated with sustained increases in alcohol- and anxiety-related emergency department visits. Disparities across age and insurance status highlight differential vulnerability and access patterns requiring targeted interventions. (*Am J Public Health*. 2026;116(6): 806–809. https://doi.org/10.2105/AJPH.2026.308456)

AJPH June 2026, Vol. 116, No. 6

Hurricane Helene caused unprecedented destruction in the Appalachian region of Western North Carolina in September 2024, resulting in 108 fatalities and catastrophic infrastructure damage that isolated entire communities.[1] Even before Hurricane Helene, the Appalachian region faced unique challenges, including persistent socioeconomic and health disparities, elevated youth suicide risk and substance misuse, and limited access to behavioral health services.[2–4] Previous hurricanes and extreme floods across the Southeast have demonstrated sustained increases in depression, anxiety, and substance use disorder,[5–6] yet little is known about the mental health and substance use consequences of disasters in rural Appalachia, an inland location with pronounced health disparities.

We sought to quantify temporal changes in mental health and substance use emergency department (ED) utilization following Hurricane Helene in Western North Carolina and identify disparities across vulnerable populations.

METHODS

We conducted a cross-sectional analysis using North Carolina Disease Event Tracking and Epidemiologic Collection Tool ED surveillance data. We analyzed ED visits for residents of 19 Western North Carolina counties most affected by Hurricane Helene.[7] We identified outcomes using *ICD-10* (*International Classification of Diseases, 10th Revision*. Geneva, Switzerland: World Health Organization; 1992) codes in any diagnostic position (primary or secondary) and included mental health (*ICD-10*: F01–F99) and substance use disorder (*ICD-10*: F10–F19) with associated subdisorders (Table A, available as a supplement to the online version of this article at http://www.ajph.org).

We based recovery periods on Hurricane Helene's September 26, 2024, landfall and regional recovery context: immediate impact (September 26–October 10, 2024; weeks 1–2 after landfall), early recovery (October 11–November 15, 2024; weeks 3–7), and short-term recovery (November 16–December 31, 2024; weeks 8–14). The reference period spanned the corresponding calendar dates in 2023 (September 26–December 31). We calculated incidence rate ratios (IRRs) comparing recovery periods to the baseline using Poisson regression, with negative binomial models for overdispersed data (dispersion > 2.0). Models included county-level demographics derived from the American Community Survey (proportions of those aged ≥ 65 years, female, Black, Hispanic, and uninsured or covered by Medicaid), temporal controls (month and day of the week), and log (person-time) as an offset. We assessed effect modification using individual-level patient characteristics (age, sex, insurance status) and county-level measures (rurality, derived from American Community Survey data), employing interaction terms with counties dichotomized at median values. We set significance at $P < .05$. We used R version 4.2.3 (RStudio, Boston, MA) for all analyses.

RESULTS

We analyzed 24 981 mental health ED visits (including 17 762 substance use visits) across both study periods. The 2024 posthurricane period included 12 834 visits and the 2023 reference period included 12 147 (Table B, available as a supplement to the online version of this article at http://www.ajph.org).

Main Effects

Alcohol-related ED visits increased across all post–Hurricane Helene periods compared with 2023 (immediate: IRR = 1.35; 95% confidence interval [CI] = 1.14, 1.60; early: IRR = 1.47; 95% CI = 1.31, 1.65; short-term: IRR = 1.36; 95% CI = 1.21, 1.52). Anxiety disorders increased across all periods (immediate: IRR = 1.15; 95% CI = 1.02, 1.28; early: IRR = 1.12; 95% CI = 1.03, 1.21; short-term: IRR = 1.17; 95% CI = 1.09, 1.26). Mood disorders increased during early recovery (IRR = 1.13; 95% CI = 1.04, 1.23). Schizophrenia-related ED visits increased significantly during short-term recovery (IRR = 1.19; 95% CI = 1.02, 1.40), and opioid-related ED visits showed elevated point estimates that reached marginal significance (IRR = 1.21; 95% CI = 1.00, 1.45). Overall mental health, depression, posttraumatic stress disorder–, suicide-, and cannabis-related ED visits showed no significant changes (Figure 1).

Effect Modification

Counties with higher elderly ED patient populations (≥ 31.8% aged ≥ 65 years) experienced greater alcohol effects across all periods (immediate: IRR = 1.79 vs 0.96; early: IRR = 1.98 vs 1.21; short-term: IRR = 1.85 vs 1.18; interaction $P < .001$) and amplified anxiety effects (immediate: IRR = 1.42 vs 0.82; interaction $P < .001$). Counties with higher uninsured or covered by Medicaid rates (≥ 31.7%) showed lower posthurricane utilization than did counties with lower rates for alcohol- (immediate: IRR = 1.15 vs 1.59; interaction $P = .048$), anxiety- (IRR = 0.99 vs 1.31; interaction $P = .010$), and suicide- (early: IRR = 0.87 vs 1.41; interaction $P = .007$) related ED visits. Rural counties experienced greater increases in mood disorders during early recovery (IRR = 1.38 vs 1.07; interaction $P = .001$).

Counties with higher minority ED patient populations showed smaller alcohol increases (early: IRR = 1.40 vs 1.81; interaction $P = .037$; short-term: IRR = 1.29 vs 1.75; interaction $P = .009$) and mood disorder increases (early: IRR = 1.09 vs 1.33; interaction $P = .023$), but larger opioid increases during immediate impact (IRR = 1.55 vs 0.88; interaction $P = .039$). No significant modification was found regarding sex.

DISCUSSION

Our analysis reveals sustained increases in alcohol- and anxiety-related ED visits following Hurricane Helene, with marginally significant elevations in opioid- and schizophrenia-related ED visits during short-term recovery. The absence of increases in overall mental health-, posttraumatic stress disorder–, depression-, and suicide-related ED visits, contrary to disaster literature,[5–6] may reflect infrastructure-related access barriers rather than actual reduced morbidity. Widespread road closures and bridge failures that isolated entire communities likely prevented care seeking for nonacute conditions,[1,7] whereas competing survival priorities delayed mental health treatment.

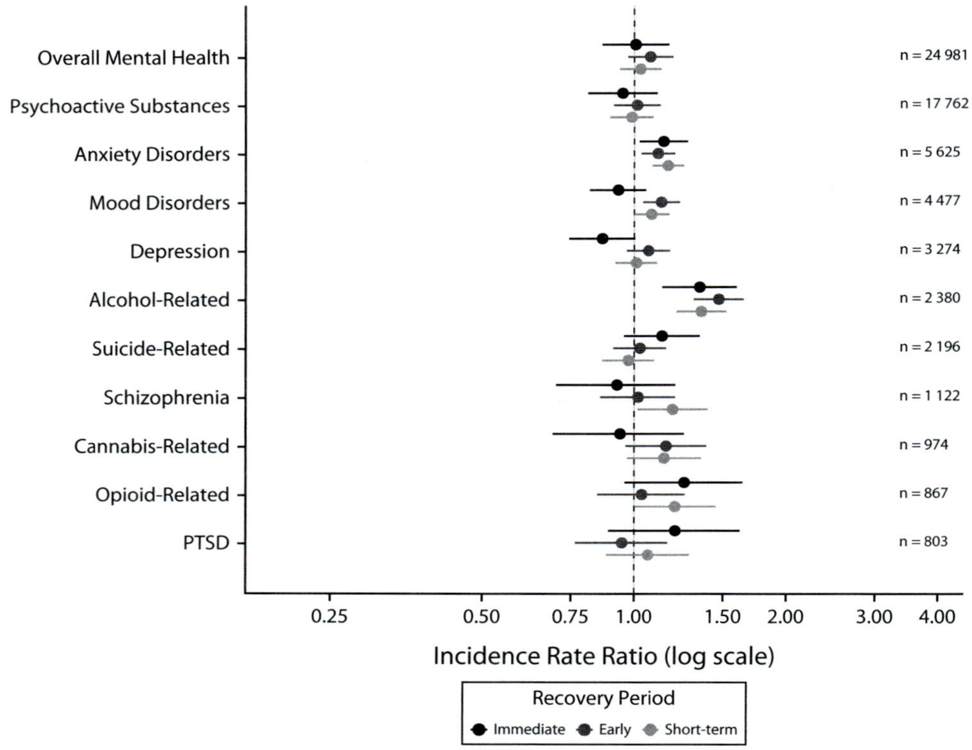

FIGURE 1— Mental Health and Substance Use ED Visits Across 3 Recovery Periods Following Hurricane Helene (2024) Compared With 2023: Western North Carolina

Note. ED = emergency department; PTSD = posttraumatic stress disorder. Black circles = immediate impact (September 26–October 10, 2024); dark gray circles = early recovery (October 11–November 15, 2024); light gray circles = short-term recovery (November 16–December 31, 2024). We analyzed ED visits for residents of the 19 Western North Carolina counties most affected by Hurricane Helene: Alleghany, Ashe, Avery, Buncombe, Cherokee, Clay, Graham, Haywood, Henderson, Jackson, Macon, Madison, McDowell, Mitchell, Polk, Swain, Transylvania, Watauga, and Yancey.

Disparities across county-level characteristics reveal differential vulnerability and access patterns. Counties with higher elderly ED populations experienced amplified alcohol and anxiety increases. By contrast, counties with higher uninsured or covered by Medicaid rates had lower posthurricane period ED utilization than did those with lower rates, suggesting that disaster-imposed access barriers (e.g., transportation and infrastructure damage) may have compounded otherwise typical utilization patterns.[8] Rural counties demonstrated greater mood disorder increases, and counties with higher minority populations showed smaller alcohol increases but larger opioid increases, indicating complex interactions between disaster exposure, health care access, housing instability, and substance use patterns requiring further investigation.

ED visits are only the most severe, acute instances requiring emergency care, substantially underestimating the population burden of mental health and substance use effects. Less severe cases, managed in primary care or outpatient settings or left untreated, were not captured in this surveillance system. Potential biases included selection bias owing to access barriers and cultural factors, information bias related to *ICD-10* coding, and confounding by secular trends (e.g., changes in regional insurance networks). Future research can use Medicaid claims data to track shifts in utilization across care settings, including primary care and outpatient behavioral health services, or employ multilevel designs that incorporate disaster impact gradients across affected and control groups to strengthen causal inference. Despite these limitations, the increases we observed in severe encounters signal a broader crisis requiring multilevel surveillance approaches beyond emergency care to capture the full spectrum of disaster mental health consequences.

PUBLIC HEALTH IMPLICATIONS

Public health officials should anticipate evolving mental health needs over the recovery period, as the Substance

Abuse and Mental Health Services Administration community disaster recovery model suggests these early increases may be only the initial phase of behavioral health effects, with subsequent surges in depression expected 6 to 9 months after Hurricane Helene during the disillusionment phase and a potential rise in posttraumatic stress disorder prevalence 18 to 24 months later as longer-term recovery challenges emerge.[9–10]

As disasters are becoming more frequent, practitioners should be aware of the recurring expressions of trauma among first responders, local officials, and community members and avoid retraumatization by incorporating trauma-informed practices in recovery.[11] Given the disproportionate impacts observed among elderly and rural populations, strategies such as community-based peer support and targeted outreach to high-risk groups will be crucial to reducing unmet needs. AJPH

ABOUT THE AUTHORS

Margaret M. Sugg, Sophia C. Ryan, and Christine Quattro are with the Department of Geography and Planning, College of Arts and Sciences, Appalachian State University, Boone, NC. Annie Preaux, Martie P. Thompson, and Adam Hege are with the Department of Public Health, Beaver College of Health Sciences, Appalachian State University. Ben Alexander-Eitzman is with the Department of Social Work, Beaver College of Health Sciences. Jennifer D. Runkle is with the North Carolina Institute for Climate Studies, North Carolina State University, Asheville.

CORRESPONDENCE

Correspondence should be sent to Maggie M. Sugg, PhD, Department of Geography and Planning, Appalachian State University, ASU Box 32066, 572 Rivers St, Boone, NC 28608 (e-mail: kovachmm@appstate.edu). Reprints can be ordered at https://www.ajph.org by clicking the "Reprints" link.

PUBLICATION INFORMATION

Full Citation: Sugg MM, Ryan SC, Preaux A, et al. Emergency department burden of mental health and substance misuse after Hurricane Helene: insights from rural Appalachia. *Am J Public Health*. 2026;116(6):806–809.

Acceptance Date: February 2, 2026.

DOI: https://doi.org/10.2105/AJPH.2026.308456

ORCID iDs:

Margaret M. Sugg https://orcid.org/0000-0002-0315-4860

Christine Quattro https://orcid.org/0000-0003-3667-5029

Ben Alexander-Eitzman https://orcid.org/0000-0002-2329-1678

Martie P. Thompson https://orcid.org/0000-0002-5879-9615

CONTRIBUTORS

M. M. Sugg conceptualized the study, conducted the statistical analyses, and drafted the brief. S. C. Ryan assisted with data processing. A. Preaux, C. Quattro, and B. Alexander-Eitzman provided feedback. M. P. Thompson and A. Hege obtained funding. J. D. Runkle contributed to the study methodology. All authors critically reviewed and approved the final version of the brief.

ACKNOWLEDGMENTS

The North Carolina Disease Event Tracking and Epidemiologic Collection Tool (NC DETECT) is an advanced, statewide public health surveillance system. NC DETECT is funded with federal funds by the North Carolina Division of Public Health (NC DPH), Public Health Emergency Preparedness Grant (PHEP), and managed through a collaboration between NC DPH and the University of North Carolina at Chapel Hill Department of Emergency Medicine's Carolina Center for Health Informatics (UNC CCHI). This work was also supported by the University of North Carolina Collaboration Grant (award no. 592), the National Science Foundation (C2H2 RCN collaborative research grant 2525761), and the Dogwood Health Trust (grant no. 5541).

Note. The findings and conclusions in this publication are those of the author(s) and do not necessarily represent the views of the North Carolina Department of Health and Human Services, Division of Public Health.

CONFLICTS OF INTEREST

The authors have no conflicts of interest to disclose.

HUMAN PARTICIPANT PROTECTION

This study was approved by the Appalachian State University institutional review board (protocol no. HS-25-69).

REFERENCES

1. North Carolina Office of State Budget and Management. *Hurricane Helene Recovery*. December 13, 2024. Available at: https://www.osbm.nc.gov/hurricane-helene-dna/open. Accessed March 24, 2026.
2. Krometis LA, Gohlke J, Kolivras K, Satterwhite E, Marmagas SW, Marr LC. Environmental health disparities in the central Appalachian region of the United States. *Rev Environ Health*. 2017;32(3):253–266. https://doi.org/10.1515/reveh-2017-0012
3. McGarvey EL, Leon-Verdin M, Killos LF, Guterbock T, Cohn WF. Health disparities between Appalachian and non-Appalachian counties in Virginia USA. *J Community Health*. 2011;36(3):348–356. https://doi.org/10.1007/s10900-010-9315-9
4. Sugg MM, Ryan SC, Ulrich SE, Runkle JD, Thompson MP. Structural influences on psychiatric emergency department visits among racial and ethnic minority youth in North Carolina: a neighborhood-level analysis. *Health Place*. 2024;90:103379. https://doi.org/10.1016/j.healthplace.2024.103379
5. Miller VE, Fitch KV, Swilley-Martinez ME, et al. Impact of hurricanes and floodings on mental health outcomes within the United States: a systematic review and meta-analysis. *Disaster Med Public Health Prep*. 2025;18:e335. https://doi.org/10.1017/dmp.2024.327
6. Runkle JD, Michael KD, Stevens SE, Sugg MM. Quasi-experimental evaluation of text-based crisis patterns in youth following Hurricane Florence in the Carolinas, 2018. *Sci Total Environ*. 2021;750:141702. https://doi.org/10.1016/j.scitotenv.2020.141702
7. Sugg M, Blackburn C, Ryan S, Cardwell J, Gohlke J, Runkle J. Rural–urban disparities in Hurricane Helene's disaster assistance in Western North Carolina. *J Appalach Inst Health Wellness*. 2025. Available at: https://jihhs.pubpub.org/pub/t94hm77m. Accessed March 24, 2026.
8. Ramirez-Rios D, Wallace WA, Kinsler J, Viota NM, Mendez P. Exploring post-disaster transportation barriers to health care for socially vulnerable Puerto Rican communities. 2022. Available at: https://hazards.colorado.edu/public-health-disaster-research/exploring-post-disaster-transportation-barriers-to-healthcare-of-socially-vulnerable-puerto-rican-communities. Accessed March 24, 2026.
9. DeWolfe DJ. Field manual for mental health and human service workers in major disasters. 2000. Available at: https://www.ojp.gov/ncjrs/virtual-library/abstracts/field-manual-mental-health-and-human-service-workers-major. Accessed March 24, 2026.
10. Substance Abuse and Mental Health Services Administration. Disaster preparedness, response, recovery, and mitigation. January 16, 2025. Available at: https://www.samhsa.gov/disaster-preparedness. Accessed March 24, 2026.
11. Rosenberg H, Errett NA, Eisenman DP. Working with disaster-affected communities to envision healthier futures: a trauma-informed approach to post-disaster recovery planning. *Int J Environ Res Public Health*. 2022;19(3):1723. https://doi.org/10.3390/ijerph19031723

Challenges and Opportunities in Estimating the Mortality Burden Related to Heat Exposure: Maricopa County, Arizona, 2019–2023

Heather L. Leahy, DVM, MPH, Ambarish Vaidyanathan, PhD, David M. Hondula, PhD, Meaghan Batchelor, MPH, Nicole M. Jarrett, MSPH, R. Nicholas Staab, MD, Rebecca Sunenshine, MD, and Ariella P. Dale, PhD, MPH

See also Climate Change/Natural Disasters, pp. 761–813.

Objectives. To estimate the mortality burden attributable to daily mean temperatures during the heat season (April through October) in Maricopa County, Arizona.

Methods. We examined the effects of heat exposure on 126 854 deaths that occurred in Maricopa County during the 2019 to 2023 heat seasons. Using a quasi-Poisson regression with distributed lag nonlinear models, we estimated the cumulative relative risk (relative to 77°F) between population-weighted daily mean temperatures and all-cause mortality over a lag period of 3 days.

Results. At 99°F (the 95th percentile of the population-weighted daily mean temperature), we observed an 11% (95% confidence interval [CI] = 7%, 16%) increase in daily all-cause mortality relative to 77°F. Overall, 3036 (95% empirical CI = 968, 4887) deaths were attributable to heat, which is 57% more deaths than identified through epidemiological heat surveillance.

Conclusions. The mortality burden increases with increasing population-weighted daily mean temperatures, indicating that the effects of heat on mortality can be indirect and incompletely captured by routine surveillance.

Public Health Implications. Statistical approaches can help estimate the mortality burden associated with heat exposure, complementing countywide surveillance efforts that provide actionable insights into enhancing heat prevention strategies. (*Am J Public Health*. 2026;116(6):810–813. https://doi.org/10.2105/AJPH.2026.308443)

AJPH June 2026, Vol. 116, No. 6

In Maricopa County, Arizona, there was a yearly average of 120 days with maximum temperatures of 100°F or higher between 2019 and 2023.[1] The Maricopa County Department of Public Health (MCDPH) describes such frequently high and prolonged temperatures as the heat season, usually from April 1 through October 31. In 2006, the MCDPH deployed a heat surveillance system to track heat-related deaths, characterize trends, and provide insight for heat relief efforts. Heat-related deaths have increased steadily since the introduction of the system, with 645 deaths reported in 2023.[2]

The Maricopa County Office of the Medical Examiner investigates and certifies specific deaths, which is how most heat-related deaths are ascertained.[2,3] The office conducts comprehensive examinations, assessing autopsy findings, environmental factors, heat mitigation efforts, and risk factors for increased heat sensitivity to determine whether a death can be categorized as heat related.[2] The MCDPH receives reports on these investigations and gathers additional information from the decedent death certificates.

The MCDPH and the Office of the Medical Examiner continuously strive to improve the capturing and reporting of heat-related deaths. However, the system relies on physician-certified cause of death, allowing for the possibility of unrecognized and therefore uncounted heat-related deaths.[4] Death certificates lack consistent practices for when heat should be listed, and identifying the correct sequence of causes leading to death can be challenging.[5] For example, deaths indirectly related to heat (e.g., people dying of a heart attack in the hospital after overexerting themselves outside the day before) might be missed during the ascertainment and investigation of heat-related deaths.

The MCDPH sought to estimate the total number of heat-attributable deaths, directly and indirectly caused by heat, to enhance local public health actions and support increased local and statewide resources. We investigated the association between temperature and mortality in Maricopa County by estimating heat-attributable deaths occurring during the 2019 to 2023 heat seasons (April 1 through October 31).

METHODS

Death certificates for all people who died in Maricopa County during the 2019 to 2023 heat seasons were obtained from the Arizona Electronic Death Registry System. To account for pandemic-related mortality, we excluded deaths listing COVID-19 as an underlying or contributing cause. Remaining deaths were aggregated by date of death to generate daily all-cause mortality counts for the county.

Temperature data were obtained from DAYMET, a gridded, statistical model of surface weather conditions (https://daymet.ornl.gov/web_services). Daily minimum and maximum temperatures were averaged within Maricopa County census tracts (obtained from the 2021 US Census) and population weighted to produce county-level daily mean temperatures. Countywide aggregates of daily 24-hour average concentrations of particulate matter of 10 microns or less (PM_{10}) were obtained from the National Syndromic Surveillance Program.

We applied a quasi-Poisson distributed lag nonlinear model to estimate the association between population-weighted daily mean temperature and all-cause mortality.[4,6] Results are summarized as relative risks (RRs) in comparison with 77°F and estimated over a 3-day lag period to account for the delayed effects of heat.[7] The first reported heat-related death during 2019 to 2023 occurred at an average temperature of 77°F. Our selection of this statistical framework is consistent with previous heat-health studies estimating the excess burden associated with heat exposure.[6–8] The model included a linear function for PM_{10}[9] and an indicator for state holidays, day of the week, and year. We controlled for seasonality and interannual time trends using a natural cubic spline with 4 degrees of freedom per year.[7,8]

We calculated daily numbers of heat-attributable deaths by multiplying the attributable fraction from the temperature-specific relative risks by the baseline number of all-cause deaths observed over the 3-day lag period.[10,11] The total heat burden was estimated by summing daily heat-attributable deaths.

We performed sensitivity analyses evaluating heat-attributable mortality estimates under alternative model specifications (e.g., inclusion of COVID-19 deaths and variations in temperature reference points and lag days). All analyses were conducted with the ArcGIS Pro and R version 4.4.2 (R Foundation for Statistical Computing, Vienna, Austria) dlnm and attrdl packages.[10,12]

RESULTS

A total of 126 854 all-cause deaths (excluding deaths from COVID-19) occurred during the 2019 to 2023 heat seasons in Maricopa County (Table 1).

Mortality risks increased with increases in population-weighted daily mean temperatures (Figure A, available as a supplement to the online version of this article at http://www.ajph.org). At 99°F (the 95th percentile of the population-weighted daily mean temperature), we observed an 11% (95% confidence interval [CI] = 7%, 16%) increase in daily all-cause mortality relative to 77°F. Our model estimated that 2.39% (95% empirical CI = 0.86%, 3.93%) of deaths were attributable to heat, corresponding to an estimated total of 3036 (95% empirical CI = 968, 4887) deaths (Table 1). The model identified 57% more deaths than identified by the MCDPH heat surveillance system across the 5-year heat season (n = 1931 heat-related deaths).

Estimates were largely robust across our sensitivity analyses, with the largest changes observed when the lag structure was modified (Table A, available as a supplement to the online version of this article at http://www.ajph.org).

DISCUSSION

Our implementation of distributed lag nonlinear models at the local level revealed that as population-weighted daily mean temperatures increased, the risk for mortality in Maricopa County also increased. Our findings indicate that the effects of heat on mortality are greater than what is identified through local-level epidemiological surveillance by a considerable margin. As jurisdictions advocate for and allocate resources for heat relief, heat-attribution

TABLE 1— Comparison of Estimated and Reported Mortality Related to Heat Exposure: Maricopa County, Arizona, 2019–2023

	Deaths, No.[a]	Heat-Attributable Deaths From Statistical Modeling, No.[b] (95% Empirical CI)	Heat-Related Deaths From MCDPH Surveillance System, No.[c]
Total	126 854	3 036 (968, 4 887)	1 931
5-year average[d]	25 371	607 (194, 977)	386

Note. CI = confidence interval; MCDPH = Maricopa County Department of Public Health.
[a]Number of all-cause, non-COVID deaths among Maricopa County residents reported to the Arizona Electronic Death Registry System during the heat seasons (April 1 through October 31) of 2019 to 2023.
[b]Estimated cumulative heat-attributable fraction multiplied by baseline all-cause deaths observed over the 3-day lag period.
[c]Reported heat-related deaths from the MCDPH heat surveillance system as reflected in the 2023 heat-related death report (https://www.maricopa.gov/ArchiveCenter/ViewFile/Item/5820).
[d]Numbers were rounded up after dividing by 5 to achieve the average over the project period.

methods can offer valuable insights into the magnitude and timing of heat-related mortality. However, these approaches do not provide the geographic or demographic specificity that local heat surveillance systems can offer, which is crucial for ensuring that limited resources are directed toward heat relief strategies with the greatest potential benefit.

Our analysis highlights multiple strengths of statistical attribution methods in health outcome studies, especially when they are paired with local time-series data. These models capture complex exposure–response relationships, including nonlinear and lagged effects, with our model showing increased mortality at higher temperatures concentrated within 0 to 2 days of lagged exposure (Figure B, available as a supplement to the online version of this article at http://www.ajph.org). Flexibility in accounting for temporal confounders, such as seasonal trends or day-of-week effects, can also be included. Finally, changes in heat-attributable deaths can be explored at different points during the heat season (Figure C, available as a supplement to the online version of this article at http://www.ajph.org), supporting enhanced public health action in near- and long-term phases.

The complexity of statistical attribution can be a limitation for its application in local or state public health work. The models are sensitive to modeling choices, such as lag time selection and basis functions,[6] and sensitivity analyses are important in understanding the impact of these choices. The statistical expertise required might be outside the scope of routine public health work. The granularity of these modeling insights is limited, and they lack specificity regarding populations that might be more affected than others by heat. This includes the geographic location of deaths, which emphasizes the importance of continued epidemiological surveillance. Furthermore, although these models can capture associations between exposures and outcomes, causation cannot be established, and estimates might not fully account for unmeasured or unknown confounders.

PUBLIC HEALTH IMPLICATIONS

Statistical heat-attribution methods can help estimate mortality effects, complementing existing surveillance efforts to provide actionable insights for enhancing heat prevention strategies. Specifically, we were able to estimate the effects of increasing daily average temperatures on mortality in Maricopa County, advancing the work of local, state, federal, and nongovernmental partners. Investments in heat–health interventions by agencies and partners can be more effective when informed by such analyses and can possibly extend beyond what heat mortality surveillance alone can achieve. AJPH

ABOUT THE AUTHORS

At the time of this study, Heather L. Leahy was with the Maricopa County Department of Public Health, Phoenix, AZ; the Arizona Department of Health Services, Phoenix; and the Epidemic Intelligence Service, Centers for Disease Control and Prevention, Atlanta, GA. Ambarish Vaidyanathan is with the National Center for Environmental Health, Centers for Disease Control and Prevention, Atlanta, GA, and the School of Civil and Environmental Engineering, Georgia Institute of Technology, Atlanta. David M. Hondula is with the School of Geographical Sciences and Urban Planning, Arizona State University, Tempe. At the time of this study, Meaghan Batchelor and Rebecca Sunenshine were with the Maricopa County Department of Public Health, Phoenix, AZ. Nicole M. Jarrett, R. Nicholas Staab, and Ariella P. Dale are with the Maricopa County Department of Public Health, Phoenix, AZ.

CORRESPONDENCE

Correspondence should be sent to Heather L. Leahy, DVM, MPH, 4041 N Central Ave, Phoenix, AZ 85012 (e-mail: heather.leahy@maricopa.gov). Reprints can be ordered at https://www.ajph.org by clicking the "Reprints" link.

PUBLICATION INFORMATION

Full Citation: Leahy HL, Vaidyanathan A, Hondula DM, et al. Challenges and opportunities in estimating the mortality burden related to heat exposure: Maricopa County, Arizona, 2019–2023. *Am J Public Health*. 2026;116(6):810–813.

Acceptance Date: January 7, 2026.

DOI: https://doi.org/10.2105/AJPH.2026.308443

ORCID iDs:

Heather L. Leahy https://orcid.org/0009-0003-9902-9742

Ambarish Vaidyanathan https://orcid.org/0000-0002-7427-5256

Meaghan Batchelor https://orcid.org/0009-0000-0872-3869

Rebecca Sunenshine https://orcid.org/0000-0002-0880-1422

Ariella P. Dale https://orcid.org/0000-0003-1891-919X

CONTRIBUTORS

H. L. Leahy contributed to the acquisition, analysis, and interpretation of data for the work; assisted in conceptualizing the project; and wrote and edited the article for important intellectual content. A. Vaidyanathan, D. M. Hondula, N. M. Jarrett, and R. N. Staab contributed to the analysis and interpretation of data for the work. M. Batchelor contributed to the acquisition, analysis, and interpretation of data for the work. R. Sunenshine and A. P. Dale conceptualized the project, contributed to the analysis and interpretation of data for the work, and provided project supervision. All of the authors critically reviewed drafts.

ACKNOWLEDGMENTS

We respectfully acknowledge the individuals whose deaths are reflected in this analysis. We also thank the Maricopa County Department of Public Health Climate and Health team and the Maricopa County Office of the Medical Examiner for continued support and expertise.

Note: The findings and conclusions in this report are those of the authors and do not necessarily represent the official position of the Centers for Disease Control and Prevention.

CONFLICTS OF INTEREST

Heather L. Leahy and Ariella P. Dale received travel accommodations from the Arizona Infectious Diseases Society to present on infectious diseases in 2022 and 2024, respectively. Also, Ariella P. Dale received scholarships from the National Association of County and City Health Officials and the Council of State and Territorial Epidemiologists (CSTE) to attend the Integrated Foodborne Outbreak Response and Management western regional meeting in 2023 and the CSTE annual meeting in 2025, respectively. R. Nicholas Staab and Ariella P. Dale serve on the Arizona Department of Health Services Human Subjects Review Board. The remaining authors report no conflicts of interest.

HUMAN PARTICIPANT PROTECTION

This study was reviewed by the Centers for Disease Control and Prevention (CDC), deemed not to be human participant research, and conducted in a manner consistent with applicable federal law and CDC policy.

REFERENCES

1. National Weather Service. NOWData: NOAA Online Weather Data. Available at: https://www.weather.gov/wrh/climate?wfo=psr. Accessed February 10, 2025.
2. Maricopa County. Heat reports. Available at: https://www.maricopa.gov/1858/Heat-Surveillance. Accessed February 10, 2025.
3. Arizona State Legislature. Reporting of certain deaths; failure to report; violation; classification. Available at: https://www.azleg.gov/viewdocument/?docName=https://www.azleg.gov/ars/11/00593.htm. Accessed April 8, 2025.
4. Weinberger KR, Harris D, Spangler KR, Zanobetti A, Wellenius GA. Estimating the number of excess deaths attributable to heat in 297 United States counties. *Environ Epidemiol.* 2020;4(3):e096. https://doi.org/10.1097/EE9.0000000000000096
5. Shen T, Howe HL, Alo C, Moolenaar RL. Toward a broader definition of heat-related death: comparison of mortality estimates from medical examiners' classification with those from total death differentials during the July 1995 heat wave in Chicago, Illinois. *Am J Forensic Med Pathol.* 1998;19(2):113–118. https://doi.org/10.1097/00000433-199806000-00003
6. Gasparrini A, Armstrong B, Kenward MG. Distributed lag non-linear models. *Stat Med.* 2010;29(21):2224–2234. https://doi.org/10.1002/sim.3940
7. Metzger KB, Ito K, Matte TD. Summer heat and mortality in New York City: how hot is too hot? *Environ Health Perspect.* 2010;118(1):80–86. https://doi.org/10.1289/ehp.0900906
8. Vaidyanathan A, Saha S, Vicedo-Cabrera AM, et al. Assessment of extreme heat and hospitalizations to inform early warning systems. *Proc Natl Acad Sci U S A.* 2019;116(12):5420–5427. https://doi.org/10.1073/pnas.1806393116
9. Crooks JL, Cascio WE, Percy MS, Reyes J, Neas LM, Hilborn ED. The association between dust storms and daily non-accidental mortality in the United States, 1993–2005. *Environ Health Perspect.* 2016;124(11):1735–1743. https://doi.org/10.1289/EHP216
10. Gasparrini A, Leone M. Attributable risk from distributed lag models. *BMC Med Res Methodol.* 2014;14(1):55. https://doi.org/10.1186/1471-2288-14-55
11. Greenland S. Interval estimation by simulation as an alternative to and extension of confidence intervals. *Int J Epidemiol.* 2004;33(6):1389–1397. https://doi.org/10.1093/ije/dyh276
12. Gasparrini A. Distributed lag linear and non-linear models in R: the package dlnm. Available at: https://pmc.ncbi.nlm.nih.gov/articles/PMC3191524. Accessed February 10, 2025.

Weakening Air Quality Standards Risks Reversing Health Gains

Shreepada Tripathy, MD, MBA, MS-SA

Recent decades of air quality regulation have led to substantial declines in ambient fine particulate matter ($PM_{2.5}$) across the United States, contributing to improvements in population health. However, recent actions to reconsider or weaken national $PM_{2.5}$ standards threaten to reverse these gains. In this analytic essay, I argue that air quality regulation functions as a foundational public health intervention and a form of primary prevention, rather than solely as an environmental or industrial policy. Drawing on epidemiological evidence, I examine how reductions in $PM_{2.5}$ exposure have produced uneven health benefits across communities.

Structural disadvantage, including racial segregation and socioeconomic deprivation, has limited improvements in air quality and amplified vulnerability to pollution-related harms. Weakening $PM_{2.5}$ standards risks widening existing health inequities, increasing preventable morbidity, and shifting avoidable burdens onto public health and health care systems, particularly those serving marginalized populations.

As policymakers consider changes to air quality regulation, public health impacts and environmental justice considerations must be central to decision-making. Maintaining strong $PM_{2.5}$ standards is a critical preventive strategy for sustaining population health gains and protecting the communities at greatest risk. (*Am J Public Health*. 2026;116(6):814–818. https://doi.org/10.2105/AJPH.2026.308533)

AJPH June 2026, Vol. 116, No. 6

Recent progress in reducing ambient fine particulate matter ($PM_{2.5}$) in the United States faces renewed uncertainty. In March 2025, the US Environmental Protection Agency (EPA) proposed reconsidering the strengthened annual $PM_{2.5}$ standard, potentially weakening protections.[1]

AIR QUALITY REGULATION AS PUBLIC HEALTH POLICY

Over the past 2 decades, air quality regulation in the United States has quietly functioned as one of the nation's most consequential population health interventions.[2] Federal standards governing $PM_{2.5}$ have driven substantial reductions in ambient air pollution since the mid-2000s, coinciding with improvements in respiratory health, cardiovascular outcomes, and life expectancy.[3,4] Specifically, the EPA regulates $PM_{2.5}$ through the National Ambient Air Quality Standards, which were established under the Clean Air Act to protect public health with an adequate margin of safety. In February 2024, following a scientific review of the health evidence, the EPA strengthened the annual $PM_{2.5}$ National Ambient Air Quality Standards by lowering the allowable concentration from 12 μg/m^3 to 9 μg/m^3, reflecting growing evidence that adverse health effects occur even at relatively low levels of particulate exposure.[5] These gains, although rarely framed as public health successes, reflect the cumulative effects of regulatory decisions that reshaped exposure patterns across communities nationwide.

The proposal has reignited debate about environmental regulation, economic priorities, and how best to protect public health. Although often characterized as environmental or industrial policy disputes, such decisions carry direct consequences for population health, health care utilization, and the costs borne by health systems and public payers.

Accumulating epidemiological evidence indicates that $PM_{2.5}$ exposure remains harmful even at concentrations below previous regulatory thresholds, raising questions about the adequacy of existing standards.[6] As national exposure levels have declined, the health relevance of incremental changes in particulate pollution has become increasingly apparent, particularly for populations with heightened vulnerability owing to age, underlying health conditions, or structural disadvantage.[7]

Importantly, the health gains associated with cleaner air have not been shared equally. Communities characterized by higher poverty, racial segregation, and limited political capital have experienced smaller improvements in air quality and continue to face disproportionate exposure to $PM_{2.5}$.[8] These patterns suggest that air quality regulation has operated not only as a population health intervention but also as a mechanism shaping health equity.

In this analytic essay, I argue that air quality regulation should be understood as a core component of health policy and a fundamental strategy for primary prevention. Drawing on established epidemiological evidence, I examine how decisions about $PM_{2.5}$ standards shape population health, health system performance, and equity. I focus on the risks posed by $PM_{2.5}$ deregulation, emphasizing how weakening protections may undermine previous public health gains while disproportionately affecting already vulnerable communities.

WHAT WE KNOW ABOUT $PM_{2.5}$ AND HEALTH TODAY

The scientific case linking $PM_{2.5}$ to adverse health outcomes is extensive and well established. Early regulatory efforts were driven by evidence connecting higher concentrations of particulate pollution to respiratory and cardiovascular morbidity and premature mortality.[9,10] Over time, as regulatory standards tightened and ambient concentrations declined, a key policy question emerged: whether a threshold exists below which $PM_{2.5}$ exposure no longer poses meaningful health risks or whether harms persist even at the lower exposure levels now experienced by much of the US population.[11] A growing body of epidemiological evidence suggests that no clear threshold exists.

These relationships have been observed across diverse geographic settings and study designs, lending confidence to their robustness. Importantly, many of these studies identify harmful effects at $PM_{2.5}$ concentrations below previous national standards, suggesting that regulatory compliance does not equate to the absence of risk.[12]

A large body of epidemiological evidence, including studies of older adult populations, such as national Medicare cohorts, demonstrates that $PM_{2.5}$ exposure is associated with increased mortality and cardiopulmonary disease even at relatively low concentrations.[13] Evidence from pediatric populations is also compelling. Children are more susceptible to the respiratory effects of air pollution, and pediatric asthma has emerged as a sensitive indicator of pollution-related harm.[14] Recent analyses linking daily $PM_{2.5}$ exposure to asthma hospital admissions demonstrate that even modest short-term increases in particulate matter are associated with a higher risk of hospitalization.[15] These findings underscore the relevance of air quality regulation for conditions that drive preventable emergency department visits and inpatient utilization.

Beyond acute events, long-term exposure to $PM_{2.5}$ has been associated with reduced life expectancy and increased risk of chronic disease.[3] Studies examining changes in ambient $PM_{2.5}$ over time show that sustained reductions in particulate pollution correspond with gains in population longevity.[16] Notably, these associations persist at relatively low average concentrations, reinforcing the conclusion that further improvements in air quality continue to yield meaningful health benefits.

Recent work has also highlighted temporal patterns in $PM_{2.5}$-related health effects, suggesting that exposure timing matters. Short-term spikes in particulate matter, even against a backdrop of declining annual averages, can precipitate acute health events.[17] This dynamic underscores a limitation of regulatory frameworks that focus primarily on annual mean concentrations while underappreciating the health implications of day-to-day variability.

Taken together, the evidence indicates that $PM_{2.5}$ remains a consequential determinant of health at current exposure levels. The question facing policymakers is therefore not whether particulate pollution is harmful but how much risk society is willing to accept and how much of that risk regulated industries are permitted to externalize onto the public. As national standards are reconsidered, it is essential to recognize that even incremental increases in allowable $PM_{2.5}$ concentrations may translate into measurable increases in asthma morbidity, cardiovascular events, and premature mortality, outcomes that directly implicate the health care system.

UNEQUAL BENEFITS FROM CLEANER AIR

Although national declines in $PM_{2.5}$ exposure are a major public health

AJPH June 2026, Vol. 116, No. 6

success, these improvements have not been experienced uniformly across communities. Aggregate reductions in air pollution obscure substantial variation in exposure trends, with structurally disadvantaged communities often seeing smaller gains, or persistently elevated levels, of particulate matter.[7,18] As a result, the health benefits of cleaner air have accrued unevenly, reinforcing existing disparities rather than alleviating them.

A substantial body of research demonstrates that communities with higher poverty rates, greater racial and ethnic segregation, and limited political influence are more likely to be located near pollution sources, such as highways, industrial facilities, and freight corridors; yet these same communities are often distant from regulatory monitoring stations, meaning localized pollution increases may not be captured by existing monitoring networks.[19] These structural conditions shape baseline exposure and constrain the extent to which national regulatory improvements translate into meaningful reductions in $PM_{2.5}$. Even as national averages decline, relative differences between communities frequently persist.

This unequal distribution of exposure improvements has direct implications for health equity. Populations that experienced the smallest gains in air quality are often those with higher baseline vulnerability owing to comorbid conditions, limited access to preventive care, and greater reliance on safety net health systems.[20] Continued exposure to $PM_{2.5}$ in these settings compounds existing disadvantages, contributing to higher rates of asthma morbidity, cardiovascular disease, and premature mortality. Evidence linking $PM_{2.5}$ exposure to health outcomes suggests that these disparities are not merely theoretical. In such contexts, even modest increases in $PM_{2.5}$ may produce disproportionate health impacts, reflecting both higher exposure and heightened susceptibility.

These patterns are not the result of individual behavior or residential choice. They reflect historical and ongoing processes, including zoning, housing policy, transportation planning, and disinvestment, that have concentrated environmental hazards in specific neighborhoods.[8] Although national air quality standards have reduced overall pollution levels, they have not fully addressed the conditions that sustain exposure disparities.

Viewed through this lens, air quality regulation has functioned as a partial and uneven equity intervention. Proposals to weaken $PM_{2.5}$ standards risk exacerbating these inequities by allowing pollution levels to rise most in areas already experiencing higher baseline exposure and vulnerability, threatening to widen existing gaps in health outcomes.

WHAT DEREGULATION MEANS FOR HEALTH SYSTEMS

Evidence linking short-term increases in $PM_{2.5}$ to acute health events suggests that even modest relaxations of regulatory standards could translate into meaningful increases in health care utilization. Many health conditions frequently require urgent evaluation and inpatient treatment, placing immediate demands on emergency departments and hospitals.

The burden of increased utilization would not be distributed evenly across the health care system. Safety net providers, public hospitals, and Medicaid-serving institutions are disproportionately located in communities with higher baseline pollution exposure and greater social vulnerability.[21] These providers are therefore more likely to experience the downstream effects of increased $PM_{2.5}$ exposure, including higher uncompensated care, staffing strain, and capacity constraints.[22] For health systems operating with limited financial flexibility, such increases may exacerbate existing challenges in maintaining access and quality.

From a financing perspective, environmental deregulation is a shift in costs rather than a true reduction. Although loosening air quality standards may reduce compliance costs for regulated industries, the resulting health impacts generate expenses borne by patients, health systems, and public payers. Medicaid programs are likely to absorb a substantial share of these costs, given their role in covering populations at higher risk for pollution-related illness.[23] In this sense, deregulation externalizes health care costs while obscuring their connection to upstream policy decisions.

Health systems increasingly operate under payment models that emphasize prevention, population health, and cost containment.[24] Rising pollution-related morbidity runs counter to these goals, undermining efforts to reduce avoidable utilization and improve outcomes. Moreover, once environmental exposures occur, health systems have limited capacity to mitigate their effects, underscoring the importance of regulatory protections that prevent harm before it reaches the clinical setting.

Recognizing air quality regulation as a determinant of health system performance reframes debates about $PM_{2.5}$ standards. Decisions about allowable pollution levels shape not only environmental conditions but also patterns of health care demand, financial risk, and equity within the health sector. As regulatory protections are reconsidered, these health system implications should be made explicit in policy discussions about air quality standards, which have historically weighed public health benefits against economic and industrial compliance costs but often overlook the downstream effects on health systems.

POLICY IMPLICATIONS

Debates on air quality regulation are often framed as technical disputes about environmental standards or economic trade-offs. However, the evidence linking $PM_{2.5}$ exposure to adverse health outcomes makes clear that these decisions are, at their core, health policy choices. Regulatory standards governing ambient particulate matter shape patterns of disease, health care utilization, and health equity across the United States. Recognizing this connection is essential as policymakers reconsider the future of $PM_{2.5}$ regulation.

The past 2 decades demonstrate that air quality regulation can deliver substantial population health benefits. At the same time, these benefits have not been evenly distributed, with structurally disadvantaged communities experiencing smaller improvements in exposure and continuing to bear disproportionate health burdens. Regulatory decisions that permit higher levels of particulate pollution risk reinforcing these inequities while eroding previous public health gains.

From a health system perspective, weakening $PM_{2.5}$ standards is likely to increase demand for emergency and inpatient care, shifting avoidable costs to health systems and public payers. Safety net providers and Medicaid programs are particularly vulnerable to these downstream effects. As health care financing increasingly emphasizes prevention and value, environmental policies that increase pollution-related morbidity run counter to broader efforts to improve population health and control costs.

These considerations suggest several implications for policy deliberations. First, evaluations of proposed changes to air quality standards should explicitly incorporate health equity and health system impacts, examining not only aggregate health benefits and compliance costs but also the distribution of pollution-related harms and the capacity of local health systems to absorb them. Second, health sector stakeholders, including clinicians, health system leaders, and public payers, should have a clearer and more consistent role in discussions about environmental regulation. Advisory and regulatory deliberations should include clinicians and scientists with expertise in pollution-related health effects, given their responsibility for managing the downstream clinical consequences of air pollution. Finally, maintaining strong $PM_{2.5}$ standards should be viewed as a preventive health investment and a core form of primary prevention, which are essential to sustaining progress in population health rather than as an isolated environmental mandate. Reinforcing this perspective will require greater integration of environmental health into clinical training, public health practice, and health policy discussions. As the United States weighs potential changes to air quality regulation, the question is not whether $PM_{2.5}$ matters for health; the evidence is clear that it does. The more pressing question is whether policymakers are willing to risk reversing hard-won health gains and widening inequities by weakening protections against a well-established health hazard. Treating air quality regulation as health policy clarifies what is at stake: the prevention of avoidable disease, the protection of vulnerable communities, and the preservation of recent gains in population health. AJPH

ABOUT THE AUTHOR

Shreepada Tripathy is with the Department of Pediatrics, Southern Illinois University School of Medicine, Springfield.

CORRESPONDENCE

Correspondence should be sent to Shreepada Tripathy, 415 N Ninth St, PO Box 19635, Springfield, IL 62794 (e-mail: Stripathy55@siumed.edu). Reprints can be ordered at https://www.ajph.org by clicking the "Reprints" link.

PUBLICATION INFORMATION

Full Citation: Tripathy S. Weakening air quality standards risks reversing health gains. *Am J Public Health*. 2026;116(6):814–818.

Acceptance Date: March 12, 2026.

DOI: https://doi.org/10.2105/AJPH.2026.308533

ORCID iD:
Shreepada Tripathy https://orcid.org/0000-0002-7817-441X

ACKNOWLEDGMENTS

The author would like to thank the members of the Pediatric Academic Societies Health Policy Scholars Program for their thoughtful discussions and insights, which helped inform the development of this article.

CONFLICTS OF INTEREST

The author has no conflicts of interest to report.

HUMAN PARTICIPANT PROTECTION

This article did not involve human participants.

REFERENCES

1. Clean Air Task Force. EPA asks court to strike down fine particulate air pollution standard, threatening public health and undermining obligation under Clean Air Act. November 25, 2025. Available at: https://www.catf.us/2025/11/epa-asks-court-strike-down-fine-particulate-air-pollution-standard. Accessed March 25, 2026.
2. Fuller R, Landrigan PJ, Balakrishnan K, et al. Pollution and health: a progress update. *Lancet Planet Health*. 2022;6(6):e535–e547. https://doi.org/10.1016/S2542-5196(22)00090-0
3. Sun Y, Milando CW, Spangler KR, et al. Short term exposure to low level ambient fine

particulate matter and natural cause, cardiovascular, and respiratory morbidity among US adults with health insurance: case time series study. *BMJ*. 2024;384:e076322. https://doi.org/10.1136/bmj-2023-076322

4. Apte JS, Brauer M, Cohen AJ, Ezzati M, Pope CA III. Ambient $PM_{2.5}$ reduces global and regional life expectancy. *Environ Sci Technol Lett*. 2018; 5(9):546–551. https://doi.org/10.1021/acs.estlett.8b00360
5. US Environmental Protection Agency. National ambient air quality standards (NAAQS) for PM. 2024. Available at: https://www.epa.gov/pm-pollution/national-ambient-air-quality-standards-naaqs-pm#:~:text=On%20February%207%2C%202024%2C%20the%20EPA%20strengthened,*%20**Retaining%20the%20secondary%20annual%20PM%20standard**. Accessed March 25, 2026.
6. Marks GB. Misuse of pollution reference standards: no safe level of air pollution. *Am J Respir Crit Care Med*. 2022;205(9):984–985. https://doi.org/10.1164/rccm.202201-0160ED
7. Bravo MA, Warren JL, Leong MC, et al. Where is air quality improving, and who benefits? A study of $PM_{2.5}$ and ozone over 15 years. *Am J Epidemiol*. 2022;191(7):1258–1269. https://doi.org/10.1093/aje/kwac059
8. Hajat A, Hsia C, O'Neill MS. Socioeconomic disparities and air pollution exposure: a global review. *Curr Environ Health Rep*. 2015;2(4): 440–450. https://doi.org/10.1007/s40572-015-0069-5
9. Seaton A, MacNee W, Donaldson K, Godden D. Particulate air pollution and acute health effects. *Lancet*. 1995;345(8943):176–178. https://doi.org/10.1016/s0140-6736(95)90173-6
10. Brook RD, Rajagopalan S, Pope CA III, et al. Particulate matter air pollution and cardiovascular disease. *Circulation*. 2010;121(21):2331–2378. https://doi.org/10.1161/CIR.0b013e3181dbece1
11. Boogaard H, Crouse DL, Tanner E, et al. Assessing adverse health effects of long-term exposure to low levels of ambient air pollution: the HEI experience and what's next? *Environ Sci Technol*. 2024;58(29):12767–12783. https://doi.org/10.1021/acs.est.3c09745
12. Wang Y, Danesh Yazdi M, Wei Y, Schwartz JD. Air pollution below US regulatory standards and cardiovascular diseases using a double negative control approach. *Nat Commun*. 2024;15(1):8451. https://doi.org/10.1038/s41467-024-52117-8
13. Hao H, Wang Y, Zhu Q, et al. National cohort study of long-term exposure to $PM_{2.5}$ components and mortality in Medicare American older adults. *Environ Sci Technol*. 2023;57(17):6835–6843. https://doi.org/10.1021/acs.est.2c07064
14. Sun BZ, Gaffin JM. Recent insights into the environmental determinants of childhood asthma. *Curr Allergy Asthma Rep*. 2024;24(5):253–260. https://doi.org/10.1007/s11882-024-01140-2
15. Tripathy S. Tiny particles, big problems: $PM_{2.5}$ exposure on pediatric asthma admissions in Illinois from 2006 to 2021. *Pediatr Open Sci*. 2025; 1(4):1–8. https://doi.org/10.1542/pedsos.2025-000884
16. Fann N, Kim S, Olives C, Sheppard L. Estimated changes in life expectancy and adult mortality resulting from declining $PM_{2.5}$ exposures in the contiguous United States: 1980–2010. *Environ Health Perspect*. 2017;125(9):097003. https://doi.org/10.1289/EHP507
17. Horne BD, Joy EA, Hofmann MG, et al. Short-term elevation of fine particulate matter air pollution and acute lower respiratory infection. *Am J Respir Crit Care Med*. 2018;198(6):759–766. https://doi.org/10.1164/rccm.201709-1883OC
18. Cheeseman MJ, Ford B, Anenberg SC, et al. Disparities in air pollutants across racial, ethnic, and poverty groups at US public schools. *Geohealth*. 2022;6(12):e2022GH000672. https://doi.org/10.1029/2022GH000672
19. Di Fonzo D, Fabri A, Pasetto R. Distributive justice in environmental health hazards from industrial contamination: a systematic review of national and near-national assessments of social inequalities. *Soc Sci Med*. 2022;297:114834. https://doi.org/10.1016/j.socscimed.2022.114834
20. Hooper LG, Kaufman JD. Ambient air pollution and clinical implications for susceptible populations. *Ann Am Thorac Soc*. 2018;15(suppl 2): S64–S68. https://doi.org/10.1513/AnnalsATS.201707-574MG
21. Powell WR, Hansmann KJ, Carlson A, Kind AJH. Evaluating how safety-net hospitals are identified: systematic review and recommendations. *Health Equity*. 2022;6(1):298–306. https://doi.org/10.1089/heq.2021.0076
22. Yun BJ, Singh MK, Reznek MA, et al. Strengthening essential emergency departments: transforming the safety net. *Health Aff Sch*. 2025;3(3): qxaf044. https://doi.org/10.1093/haschl/qxaf044
23. Chen CP, Singh H, Bialowitz J, Sherman JD. The role of payers in achieving environmentally sustainable and climate resilient health care. *Health Affairs Forefront*. May 30, 2024. Available at: https://www.healthaffairs.org/content/forefront/role-payers-achieving-environmentally-sustainable-and-climate-resilient-health-care. Accessed March 25, 2026.
24. Leao DLL, Cremers HP, van Veghel D, Pavlova M, Groot W. The impact of value-based payment models for networks of care and transmural care: a systematic literature review. *Appl Health Econ Health Policy*. 2023;21(3):441–466. https://doi.org/10.1007/s40258-023-00790-z

Abortion Bans and Maternal, Pregnancy-Related, and Pregnancy-Associated Mortality in 14 US States, 2016–2023: Estimated Impacts Amid Substantial Measurement Challenges

Suzanne O. Bell, PhD, Alexander M. Franks, PhD, Amy Ozinsky, MSPH, Selena Anjur-Dietrich, PhD, Claire E. Margerison, PhD, Elizabeth A. Stuart, PhD, Avi Feller, PhD, and Alison Gemmill, PhD

Objectives. To examine the association of abortion bans with changes in maternal, pregnancy-related, and pregnancy-associated mortality.

Methods. Using national vital statistics data (2016–2023), we used a Bayesian panel model to examine maternal, pregnancy-related, and pregnancy-associated mortality in 14 US states that implemented abortion bans by the end of 2022. Models accounted for temporal trends and state-specific factors.

Results. Among the 14 states with abortion bans, there was some evidence of a potential 9.2% (95% credible interval [CI] = −1.6, 20.7) increase in the number of pregnancy-associated deaths above expectation, equivalent to 68 (95% CI = −13, 147) excess deaths; the rate was also higher than expected, with 3.3 (95% CI = −2.6, 9.0) additional deaths per 100 000 live births. Relative changes in pregnancy-related mortality were similar in magnitude but had greater uncertainty. There was no detectable increase in maternal mortality.

Conclusions. Abortion bans may be associated with an increase in pregnancy-associated and pregnancy-related mortality, although data limitations and chance variation in these rare outcomes constrain the certainty of these and other findings. (*Am J Public Health*. 2026;116(6):819–828. https://doi.org/10.2105/AJPH.2026.308465)

AJPH June 2026, Vol. 116, No. 6

The US abortion policy landscape has undergone unprecedented changes since 2021. Texas passed Senate Bill 8 in September 2021, prohibiting abortions beyond approximately 6 weeks' gestation. The following June, the Supreme Court's *Dobbs v Jackson Women's Health Organization* decision eliminated federal protections and enabled states to regulate abortion. As of early 2026, 13 states had complete abortion bans and 7 more banned abortion prior to fetal viability (approximately 22 weeks' gestation), although there has been considerable churn in these laws.[1] Evidence suggests that these policies have resulted in substantial shifts in the accessibility and mode of abortion service delivery across the United States,[2–4] with inequitable impacts on health outcomes like fertility[5–7] and infant morbidity and mortality.[8–10]

A critical question regarding the health consequences of US abortion bans is their effect on maternal health, in particular on mortality. The United States has a long-standing maternal health crisis, with higher rates of maternal deaths than peer countries and significant racial and ethnic inequities.[11,12] Three nested measures of mortality during or within 1 year of pregnancy provide complementary insight into this crisis (Figure 1). The narrowest measure is maternal mortality, the death of a person while pregnant or within 42 days of termination of pregnancy, from any cause related to or aggravated by the pregnancy or its management; there were 18.5 maternal deaths to females aged 15 to 44 years per 100 000 live births in 2023.[14] Adding late maternal deaths up to 1 year following the end of the pregnancy to maternal deaths constitutes pregnancy-related mortality, which had a rate of 28.4 deaths per 100 000 live births (see Figure 1 note).[14] Broader still, pregnancy-associated mortality encompasses any death of a person during pregnancy or within 1 year, regardless of cause, and occurs at a rate of approximately 55.2 deaths per 100 000 live births.[14] In 2023, there were 662 maternal deaths, 1019 pregnancy-related deaths, and 1979 pregnancy-associated deaths among females aged 15 to 44 years in the United States.[14]

Many have speculated that mortality among pregnant and recently pregnant individuals would increase following the imposition of abortion bans,[15] with particular concerns about impacts in states with bans that do not have health exceptions.[16] There are at least 3 mechanisms that could link abortion bans with increased mortality among pregnant people: (1) increased number of births, which have 14 times the risk of maternal death and up to 70 times the risk of pregnancy-related death than induced abortion[17,18]; (2) shifts in the composition of births toward populations experiencing the greatest structural disadvantages, which have higher rates of maternal and pregnancy-associated mortality[11,19,20]; and (3) denial of evidence-based life-saving care to pregnant people. Simulations prior to the *Dobbs* decision suggested there could be substantial impacts on maternal and pregnancy-related mortality, with greater impacts among racially minoritized groups.[21,22] Additionally, investigative reporting by news outlets has documented several cases of maternal death because of denial of evidence-based care in states with abortion bans.[23] Results from previous research on the impact of US abortion bans on fertility provide evidence of the first 2 mechanisms, as this work documented increases in live births, disproportionately among low-income and racially minoritized populations.[6]

Despite the anticipated harms of these policies on birthing people, population-level, empirical evidence on mortality among pregnant or recently pregnant individuals remains limited. Researchers interested in estimating the causal effects of these outcomes encounter several methodological challenges that complicate efforts to study these outcomes. First, maternal, pregnancy-related, and pregnancy-associated mortality are very rare

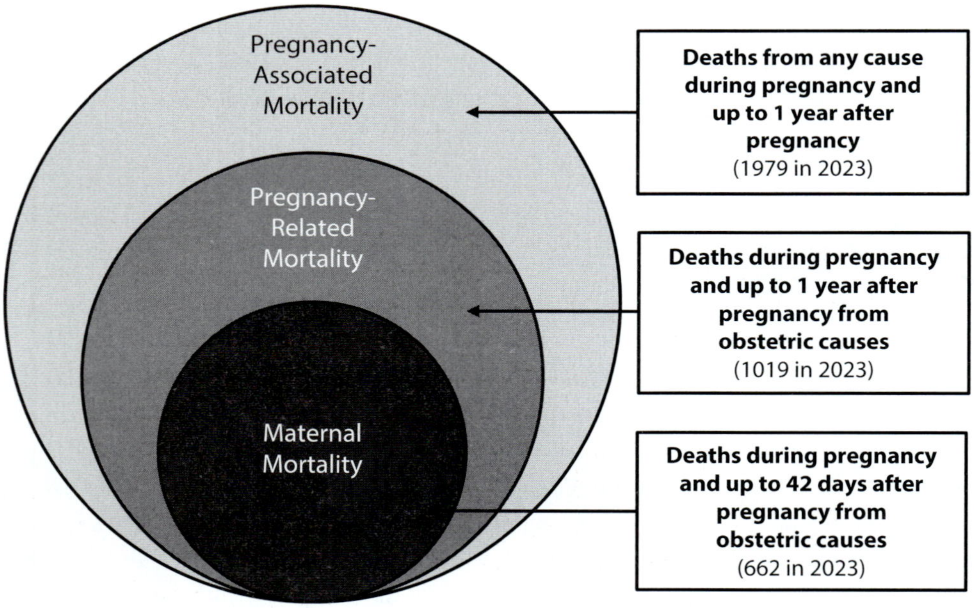

FIGURE 1— Definitions of and Relationships Between Maternal Mortality, Pregnancy-Related Mortality, and Pregnancy-Associated Mortality

Note. Counts are from CDC WONDER among females aged 15–44 years. We use this pregnancy-related mortality definition for consistency with other research but acknowledge that the Centers for Disease Control and Prevention's Pregnancy Mortality Surveillance System and state and local Maternal Mortality Review Committees apply this term based on expert review and enhanced linked data sources beyond death certificates alone to classify pregnancy-related deaths[13]; thus, our estimates are not directly comparable.

events, as previously mentioned.[13] Disaggregating these outcomes by state and over time presents substantial challenges for causal inference. Some aggregation strategies, such as grouping states by abortion ban status or using annual data, may help mitigate these issues but are not always feasible. For example, yearly aggregation requires many prepolicy intervention years. Yet, between 2003 and 2017, inconsistencies in how pregnancy status was recorded on death certificates by states introduced data artifacts.[24] Additionally, although prior research has used statistical modeling to study other rare perinatal outcomes such as infant mortality,[8–10] infant mortality is over 10 times more common than maternal mortality, making the latter far more difficult to study using similar methods.

Second, these mortality data suffer from well-documented misclassification errors and other data quality issues. In the United States and other high-income countries, maternal and pregnancy-associated deaths are frequently undercounted (i.e., false negatives) compared with gold-standard sources, like in-depth reviews of deaths to reproductive-aged women or via linkages with birth or fetal death certificate data.[25–27] At the same time, concerns have been raised about over-ascertainment (i.e., false positives) because of errors with the pregnancy checkbox on death certificates.[27,28] These include cases where a decedent is marked as pregnant or recently pregnant, but subsequent investigations find no evidence of pregnancy. These misclassification errors can be substantial and may vary by state, although the extent of this variation is not well quantified.

Third, the prepolicy period includes one of the most significant public health shocks in recent history—the COVID-19 pandemic—which had profound effects on maternal health and health care access. COVID-19 infection, particularly from later variants, has been shown to increase the risk of severe maternal complications. As a result, maternal mortality surged during the pandemic, with estimates indicating a nearly 60% increase between 2019 and 2021[20,29]; similar increases were observed for pregnancy-related mortality. Importantly, these increases were differential, with states that had the most pronounced 2021 peaks later imposing abortion bans.[30] This increase presents a major challenge for estimating counterfactual trends, as any analysis must contend with a sharp, pandemic-driven rise in maternal deaths, as well as the possibility of lingering effects beyond the maternal death spike in 2021. Such challenges may prove insurmountable given the scale and complexity of the disruption.

Given these challenges, we used a Bayesian panel data approach to estimate the association between abortion bans and maternal, pregnancy-related, and pregnancy-associated mortality in the United States, recognizing the limitations of available data. We also conducted posthoc descriptive assessments of data quality to better understand the implications of measurement issues for causal interpretation.

METHODS

This study used quarterly (e.g., January–March) counts of maternal, pregnancy-related, and pregnancy-associated deaths from restricted death certificate data compiled by the National Center for Health Statistics (NCHS) for all 50 states and the District of Columbia for 2016 through 2023.[31] Corresponding live birth counts for mortality rate calculations were drawn from the NCHS restricted birth certificate data. Per the NCHS data use agreement, we suppressed cell counts fewer than 10 in tables to protect confidentiality.

The outcomes included maternal, pregnancy-related, and pregnancy-associated mortality counts and rates, calculated as the number of deaths per 100 000 live births. We identified maternal deaths using the *International Classification of Diseases, Tenth Revision* (*ICD-10*) codes A34, O00 through O95, O98, and O99,[11] restricted to deaths among individuals aged 15 to 44 years. Pregnancy-related deaths expand the maternal death definition to include the *ICD-10* code O96.[20] Pregnancy-associated deaths were identified via the pregnancy checkbox on the death certificate, including categories 2 (not pregnant but pregnant within 42 days of death), 3 (not pregnant but pregnant 43 days to 1 year before death), and 4 (pregnant at time of death).[32] We also categorized all pregnancy-related deaths as pregnancy-associated deaths, regardless of whether the checkbox was used. To reduce the impact of COVID-19, which increased deaths during and after pregnancy, we also calculated these rates after excluding deaths attributed to COVID-19 (i.e., multiple cause of death *ICD-10* code U071).

The exposure is the imposition of a 6-week or complete abortion ban by the end of 2022, which included deaths (based on state of residence) in 14 states (Alabama, Arkansas, Georgia, Idaho, Kentucky, Louisiana, Mississippi, Missouri, Oklahoma, South Dakota, Tennessee, Texas, West Virginia, and Wisconsin). More recently imposed abortion bans were not examined as sufficient birth cohorts (and corresponding deaths) exposed to the policy were not observed during the study period. Exposure to the policy based on weeks' gestation or months since the end of the pregnancy was not possible because death certificates were not linked to birth certificates where this information is available; thus, we only used month of death to categorize exposure. Given the different hypothesized mechanisms linking abortion bans to mortality among pregnant and recently pregnant individuals and the broad timing over which these mechanisms act, we sought to minimize potential exposure misclassification by starting the exposure period at the quarter that was roughly 4 months after imposition of the abortion ban for maternal deaths and 8 months after the imposition of the abortion ban for pregnancy-related and pregnancy-associated deaths (Appendix Figure A.1, available as a supplement to the online version of this article at http://www.ajph.org).

Analyses used a Bayesian panel data approach to model counterfactual predictions of mortality counts and rates in the 14 states that imposed a complete or 6-week abortion ban. Difference-in-differences and its generalization, 2-way fixed effects, are the most common frameworks for panel data analysis of this form. These methods, however, require a parallel trends assumption that is unlikely to hold in our study. Instead, the key modeling assumption used here is that observed outcomes depend on a small number of unobserved factors, known as a low-rank factor model, which relaxes the parallel trends assumption. This approach, which is similar to prior analyses on the impact of abortion bans,[6,9] models count and rate outcomes directly and more fully captures uncertainty through partial pooling and hierarchical modeling. In states with abortion bans during exposed periods, the model for the expected outcome in the absence of abortion bans depends on the observed outcome for states with abortion bans during the preexposure period and states without abortion bans (36 remaining states and the District of Columbia) over the entire study period. Additional model details are provided in Section C of the online Appendix.

The analysis was conducted separately for counts and rates of maternal, pregnancy-related, and pregnancy-associated deaths, overall and by race and ethnicity (non-Hispanic White, non-Hispanic Black, Hispanic, and non-Hispanic other), with information obtained from death and birth certificates. Estimates are presented for all states with bans, for all states with bans excluding Texas, and for Texas separately, given its earlier exposure and evidence that Texas accounts for a large portion of the overall impact of abortion bans on population health.[6,9]

Extensive model checks were performed. Preexposure model fit was evaluated for each state, with potential anomalies identified through visual inspection. To assess whether study results could be explained by factors other than abortion bans that were influencing mortality more broadly, we conducted a placebo-in-time analysis by shifting the start of the exposure dates for each state earlier by 2 years, including data starting as early as 2012. Lastly, given concerns that use of COVID-19 cause of death codes may have been systematically different in states with and without bans, the models were also run including COVID-19 deaths to assess whether the removal of these deaths qualitatively influenced our conclusions.

All analyses were performed in R version 4.3.0 (R Foundation for Statistical Computing, Vienna, Austria) and Python version 3.11 (Python Software Foundation, Wilmington, DE). A full replication file is available at https://github.com/afranks86/maternal_mortality.

RESULTS

Appendix Figure B.2 includes maternal and all-cause pregnancy-associated mortality rates during the study period by abortion ban status and race and ethnicity. Figure 2 presents the maternal (a), pregnancy-related (b), and pregnancy-associated (c) mortality rates for states without bans, states with bans excluding Texas, and Texas, including and excluding deaths attributable to COVID-19. These data show potential increases in all mortality measures in states that banned abortion after the policies were imposed, whereas mortality rates in states that did not impose a ban stayed relatively stable. Results also illustrate the large impact of COVID-19 on these deaths, disproportionately among states that subsequently imposed an abortion ban. Efforts to remove the differential impact of COVID-19 on deaths appear insufficient, with an increase in mortality in 2021 not fully eliminated when excluding deaths with COVID-19 denoted as one of the conditions present at death.

Visual inspection of state-specific model diagnostics identified some potential anomalies in mortality data (results not shown because of data suppression requirements for counts below 10). These issues were most pronounced in Alabama, where there was a 6-month period following policy implementation that deviated sharply from historical patterns and fell below the expected range based on preexposure data ($P < .001$). In Georgia, maternal deaths also appeared lower than expected following exposure,

AJPH June 2026, Vol. 116, No. 6

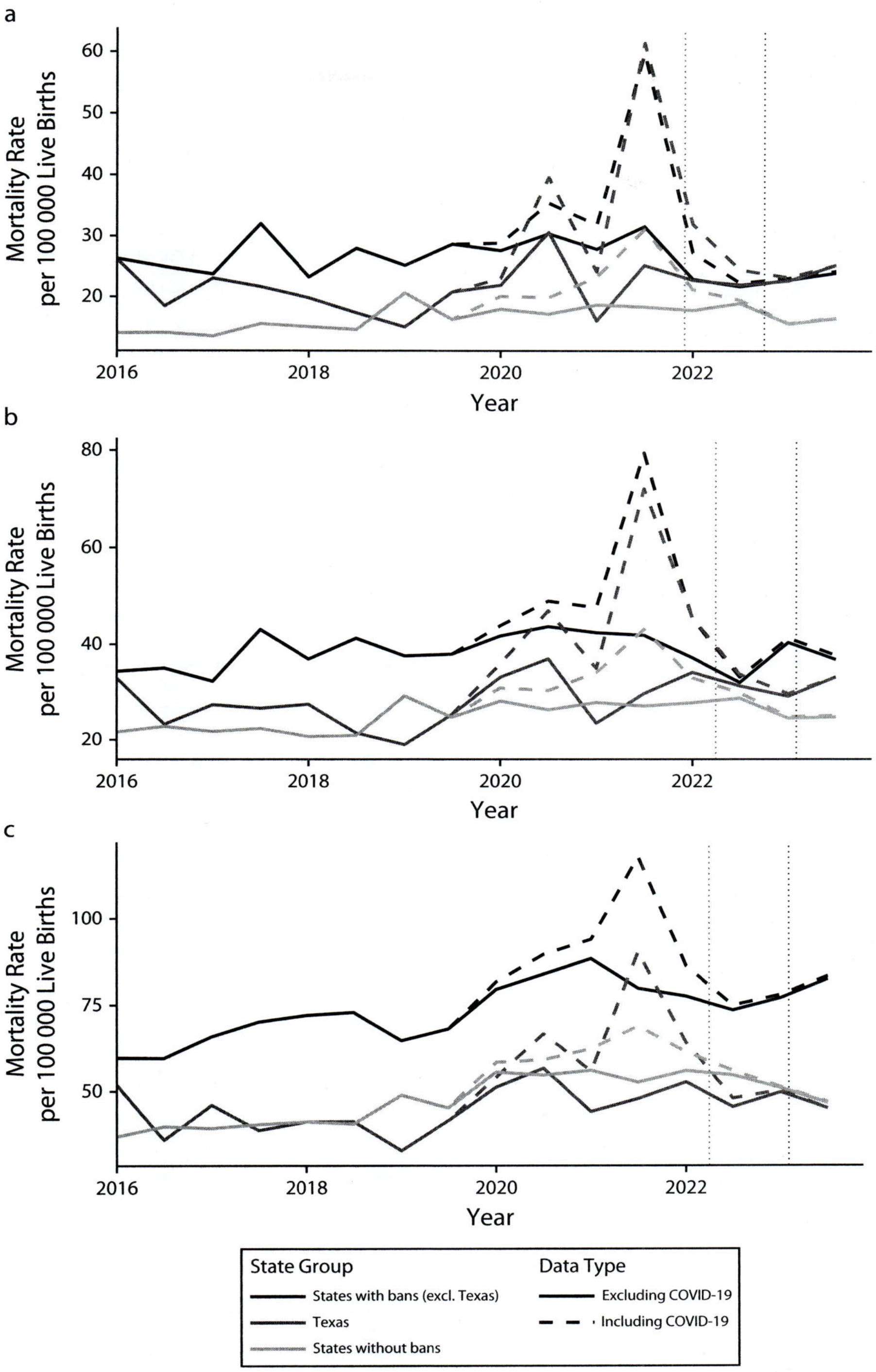

FIGURE 2— Trends in Biannual Mortality Rates per 100 000 Live Births by Abortion Ban Status, With and Without COVID-19 Attributed Deaths, for (a) Maternal Mortality, (b) Pregnancy-Related Mortality, and (c) Pregnancy-Associated Mortality: United States, 2016–2023

Note. Vertical dotted lines represent when abortion ban exposures began in Texas (dark gray) and in other states (black). Texas imposed a 6-week abortion ban the year prior to other states' bans; thus, its trendline is presented separately. Maternal mortality includes deaths during pregnancy and up to 42 days after pregnancy from obstetric causes. Pregnancy-related mortality includes deaths during pregnancy and up to 1 year after pregnancy from obstetric causes. Pregnancy-associated mortality includes deaths from any cause during pregnancy and up to 1 year after pregnancy.

although this pattern contrasts with elevated pregnancy-associated mortality during the same period.

When we used mortality data that excluded COVID-19 attributable deaths, model estimates suggested a 9.2% (95% credible interval [CI] = −1.6, 20.7) increase in the number of pregnancy-associated deaths above what would have been expected in the absence of these bans, equivalent to 68 (95% CI = −13.0, 147.0) excess deaths; the rate was also higher than expected, with 3.3 (95% CI = −2.6, 9.0) additional deaths per 100 000 live births (62.7 observed vs 59.4 expected; Figure 3 and Table 1). However, there was substantial uncertainty in these estimates. Pregnancy-associated mortality differences from expectation were similar when we excluded Texas from the model (10.9%; 95% CI = −0.9, 24.3). Estimated relative changes in the number of pregnancy-related deaths were comparable but imprecisely estimated at 9.0% (95% CI = −4.5, 23.5) above expectation; rate results estimated 1.6 (95% CI = −3.3, 6.0) additional deaths per 100 000 live births (34.6 observed vs 33.1 expected; Figure 3 and Table 1). For maternal mortality, estimates were highly uncertain and centered around no change (−0.6%; 95% CI = −14.6, 13.0), although there was weak evidence of an increase in Texas (8.4%; 95% CI = −10.5, 29.5; Figure 3). Results for all mortality outcomes stratifying by race and ethnicity were imprecise because of small counts and did not

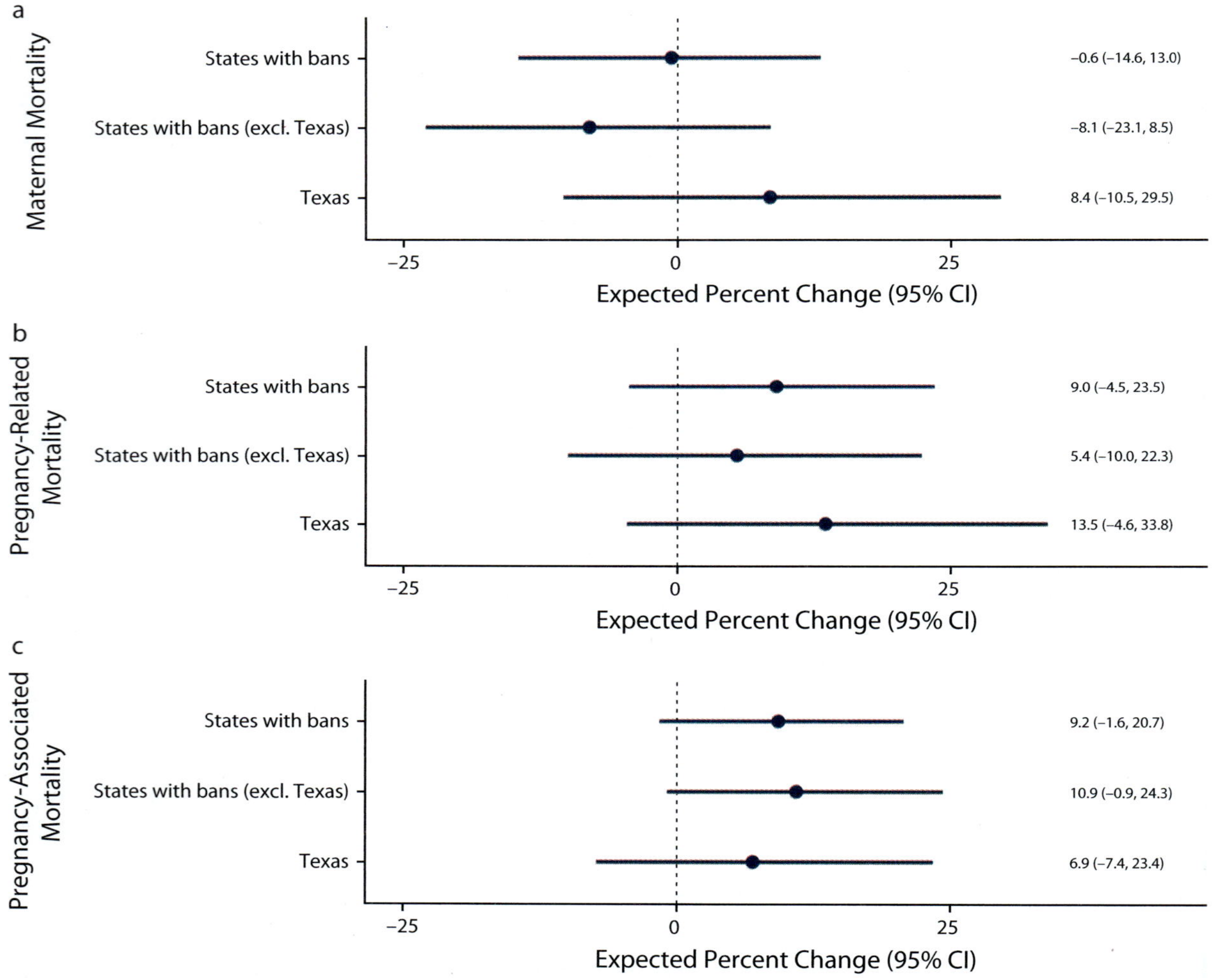

FIGURE 3— Estimated Relative Difference in the Number of Observed vs Expected Deaths in All States That Banned Abortion in Months Affected by Bans by (a) Maternal Deaths, (b) Pregnancy-Related Deaths, and (c) Pregnancy-Associated Deaths: United States, 2016–2023

Note. CI = credible interval. Maternal mortality includes deaths during pregnancy and up to 42 days after pregnancy from obstetric causes. Pregnancy-related mortality includes deaths during pregnancy and up to 1 year after pregnancy from obstetric causes. Pregnancy-associated mortality includes deaths from any cause during pregnancy and up to 1 year after pregnancy.

TABLE 1— Estimated Difference in Cumulative Observed Versus Expected Maternal, Pregnancy-Related, and Pregnancy-Associated Deaths (Count and Rate) in All US States That Banned Abortion in Months Affected by Bans: United States, 2016–2023

		Deaths			Mortality Rates (per 100 000 Live Births)			
	Births, No.	Observed, No.	Expected, No.	Expected Difference (95% CI)	Observed, No.	Expected, No.	Expected Difference (95% CI)	Expected % Change (95% CI)
Maternal mortality								
States with bans	1 690 721	397	400	−3 (−62, 49)	23.5	24.7	−1.2 (−4.2, 2.1)	−4.7 (−16.1, 9.1)
States with bans (excluding Texas)	817 451	194	212	−18 (−53, 17)	23.7	26.4	−2.7 (−6.9, 1.4)	−9.7 (−23.8, 5.3)
Texas	873 270	203	188	15 (−22, 50)	23.2	23.1	0.2 (−3.9, 4.3)	1.2 (−15.8, 20.8)
Pregnancy-related mortality								
States with bans	1 301 591	451	415	36 (−20, 93)	34.6	33.1	1.6 (−3.3, 6.0)	5.0 (−9.2, 20.0)
States with bans (excluding Texas)	618 426	232	221	11 (−24, 47)	37.5	36.8	0.7 (−5.6, 7.0)	2.2 (−14.2, 20.1)
Texas	683 165	219	194	25 (−10, 61)	32.1	29.7	2.4 (−2.9, 7.6)	8.4 (−9.0, 27.6)
Pregnancy-associated mortality								
States with bans	1 301 591	816	748	68 (−13, 147)	62.7	59.4	3.3 (−2.6, 9.0)	5.6 (−4.1, 15.9)
States with bans (excluding Texas)	618 426	490	442	48 (−4, 103)	79.2	73.3	6.0 (−2.4, 14.4)	8.4 (−3.1, 21.2)
Texas	683 165	326	306	20 (−24, 63)	47.7	46.9	0.8 (−5.4, 6.9)	2.0 (−11.0, 15.5)

Note. CI = credible interval. Count and rate results estimated from separate models. Expected mortality rates do not equal expected deaths divided by births as this model incorporates expected births in modeling the expected rate directly. Maternal mortality includes deaths during pregnancy and up to 42 days after pregnancy from obstetric causes. Pregnancy-related mortality includes deaths during pregnancy and up to 1 year after pregnancy from obstetric causes. Pregnancy-associated mortality includes deaths from any cause during pregnancy and up to 1 year after pregnancy.

suggest meaningful differences (Appendix Figure E.7).

We conducted extensive sensitivity analyses. Placebo-in-time analyses showed no change in mortality in the earlier period in states that banned abortion, with estimates centered on 0 for all outcomes (Appendix Figure E.10). As anticipated, including COVID-19 deaths worsened model fit, particularly around capturing pandemic spikes, and led to greater overall uncertainty (Appendix Figure E.8). When we excluded Alabama from the maternal mortality model because of data quality concerns, the estimated change in the number of deaths above expectation was higher than the main results (+1.9%; 95% CI = −11.0, 16.4; Appendix Figure E.9). The maternal mortality estimate among states with bans excluding Texas was attenuated when Alabama was removed (−3.2%; 95% CI = −18.4, 13.9 vs −8.1%; 95% CI = −23.1, 8.5; Appendix Figure E.9).

DISCUSSION

Study results provide suggestive evidence that pregnancy-associated and pregnancy-related mortality in states that imposed abortion bans is higher than would be expected in the absence of these policies. Specifically, there was an estimated 9% increase in the number of pregnancy-associated and pregnancy-related deaths above expectation in the 14 states examined, whereas there was weak evidence of a corresponding increase in the mortality rates. Although results are noisy, this suggests that some of the estimated increase in mortality at the population level is attributable to increases in births—as described in other research[6]—whereas the relative contribution of increased mortality risk remains less clear. There was no evidence of an impact on maternal mortality, especially after we conducted sensitivity analyses that excluded apparent data anomalies in Alabama. However, concerns over data quality and limited statistical power qualify these results.

Although the pregnancy-related and pregnancy-associated mortality results are qualitatively consistent with predictions and simulations,[15,21] study findings should be interpreted with caution because of the considerable limitations of these data. Given the rarity of maternal death in particular, this analysis struggled with statistical power to detect effects. In a 2023 simulation of the potential impact of abortion bans on maternal mortality that assumed 19 states imposed a total ban and 3 more imposed 6-week bans, the authors estimated that there would be 17 excess deaths, equivalent to a 2.7% increase above expectation.[22] Based on the uncertainty interval associated with our maternal mortality estimate, we would be quite underpowered to detect an effect of this magnitude; 95% credible intervals would exclude 0 only if there was a relative increase of 14.8%. For pregnancy-related and pregnancy-associated mortality, the smallest relative increases we could similarly detect would be 13.5% and 10.8%, respectively. This highlights the limits of what can be empirically measured at the population level for rare outcomes like these. Still, the absence of a measurable impact on maternal mortality at the population level should not be mistaken for the absence of harm, as numerous investigations have documented preventable maternal deaths in states with bans.[23]

The differences across maternal, pregnancy-related, and pregnancy-associated mortality may reflect variation in case counts as well as conceptual distinctions among these outcomes. For deaths related to obstetric causes, we did not detect a change in maternal mortality but observed suggestive increases in pregnancy-related mortality. This pattern may reflect greater statistical power because of the inclusion of late obstetric deaths, which have been increasing in the United States.[33] By contrast, pregnancy-associated mortality encompasses all causes of death during pregnancy or within 1 year of pregnancy. The majority of these deaths are still obstetric in nature, but approximately one quarter result from suicide, homicide, and drug overdose.[32] Although abortion bans are typically framed in terms of obstetric care, their effects may extend to other causes of death; emerging evidence of increased suicides among reproductive-aged women following the *Dobbs* decision highlights the need to investigate potential impacts on nonobstetric health outcomes as well.[34]

Despite the potential for these policies to worsen existing racial and ethnic disparities, we did not find strong evidence of differential impacts, although there was considerable uncertainty in our estimates. Nonetheless, states with the most restrictive abortion laws already have higher maternal mortality, particularly among non-Hispanic Black individuals, driven in part by structural barriers such as limited access to affordable health insurance and maternity care providers.[35] Additionally, a greater share of reproductive-aged racially minoritized individuals live in states with bans, making them disproportionately exposed to these policies and their impacts.[36] Investigation of potentially inequitable mortality impacts among racially minoritized populations merits additional research.

Mortality is just the "tip of the iceberg": for every maternal death, there are an estimated 60 other pregnant individuals who experience severe and potentially life-threatening complications.[37] Growing evidence suggests an increase in sepsis and hemorrhage for certain pregnancies in Texas following their 2021 6-week abortion ban,[38–40] but further research is needed to understand the broader impacts of these policies on maternal morbidity.

Limitations

This study has several limitations. First, as we document in the introduction, there are substantial data quality concerns. Although we can only identify the most pronounced data irregularities (e.g., undercounts in Alabama), there are likely others that we are not able to detect. Although maternal mortality review committees operate independently from vital statistics systems, recent decisions in states like Georgia, Idaho, and Texas to scale back maternal death review efforts raise broader concerns about the long-term commitment to maintaining robust maternal health surveillance, including the integrity of vital statistics data.[41]

Second, our COVID-19 correction is imperfect, with the remaining influence of the pandemic differentially affecting the pre-abortion-ban rates and counterfactual predictions. Additionally, identification and coding of COVID-19–related deaths may have varied over time or across states, influencing the effectiveness of our adjustment. Other factors that may influence mortality, like disruptions to care and the closure of obstetric facilities, could also have differentially affected states and contributed to divergent trends during this period. Relatedly, there were many barriers to abortion care imposed in states during the pre-abortion-ban period; these were concentrated in states that later banned abortion but were also imposed in states that did not subsequently ban abortion.[42] Our method addresses these endogeneity concerns by accounting for these prepolicy patterns in predicting expected outcomes for individual states.

Third, without linked information on weeks' gestation at birth and months since the end of the pregnancy at time of death, there are likely many deaths whose exposure is misclassified. This misclassification is likely in both directions, attenuating estimates of the true impact. Fourth, changes in how pregnancy status was recorded on death certificates during the study period may have influenced ascertainment in some states. However, our modeling approach helps account for these changes and our placebo-in-time analyses did not suggest that these changes biased our findings. Finally, because our outcomes are rare events, these analyses are underpowered to detect modest but meaningful changes, especially in analyses by race and ethnicity.

Public Health Implications

Results from this study provide suggestive evidence that abortion bans may increase pregnancy-associated and pregnancy-related mortality, although data quality concerns and random variation in these rare outcomes limit the certainty of this finding and that of the other outcome examined. The potential excess deaths occurred in states with some of the worst maternal and child health outcomes, potentially worsening existing disparities across the United States while such bans are in place.[35]

More broadly, recent efforts to address the US maternal mortality crisis have led to meaningful progress, including investments in data and surveillance, research into root causes, and the development of promising interventions.[43,44] Yet these gains remain vulnerable to policy decisions. Abortion bans and other politically driven restrictions on reproductive health can undermine momentum by introducing new risks to pregnant individuals and placing added strain on already suboptimal systems of care. Given the potential for abortion bans to worsen pregnancy-associated mortality, reinforcing maternal health as a national health priority is more urgent than ever. AJPH

ABOUT THE AUTHORS

At the time of the study, Suzanne O. Bell, Selena Anjur-Dietrich, and Amy Ozinsky were with the Department of Population, Family and Reproductive Health, Johns Hopkins Bloomberg School of Public Health, Baltimore, MD. Alexander M. Franks is with the Department of Statistics and Applied Probability, University of California, Santa Barbara. Claire E. Margerison is with the Department of Epidemiology and Biostatistics, Michigan State University, East Lansing. Elizabeth A. Stuart is with the Department of Biostatistics, Johns Hopkins Bloomberg School of Public Health, Baltimore, MD. Avi Feller is with the School of Public Policy and Department of Statistics, University of California, Berkeley. Alison Gemmill is with the Department of Epidemiology, Fielding School of Public Health, University of California, Los Angeles.

CORRESPONDENCE

Correspondence should be sent to Suzanne O. Bell, PhD, 615 N. Wolfe St, Room E4148, Baltimore, MD 21205 (e-mail: suzannebell@jhu.edu). Reprints can be ordered at http://www.ajph.org by clicking the "Reprints" link.

PUBLICATION INFORMATION

Full Citation: Bell SO, Franks AM, Ozinsky A, et al. Abortion bans and maternal, pregnancy-related, and pregnancy-associated mortality in 14 US states, 2016-2023: estimated impacts amid substantial measurement challenges. *Am J Public Health*. 2026; 116(6):819–828.

Acceptance Date: February 2, 2026.

DOI: https://doi.org/10.2105/AJPH.2026.308465

ORCID iDs:
Suzanne O. Bell https://orcid.org/0000-0002-7650-5940

Alexander M. Franks https://orcid.org/0000-0002-9329-206X

Selena Anjur-Dietrich https://orcid.org/0000-0001-5986-1858

Claire E. Margerison https://orcid.org/0000-0003-0692-2252

Elizabeth A. Stuart https://orcid.org/0000-0002-9042-8611

Avi Feller https://orcid.org/0000-0001-7319-5468

Alison Gemmill https://orcid.org/0000-0001-5879-9730

CONTRIBUTORS

S. O. Bell and A. M. Franks were co-first authors. A. Feller and A. Gemmill were co-senior authors. S. O. Bell, A. M. Franks, C. E. Margerison, E. A. Stuart, A. Feller, and A. Gemmill were responsible for the study conceptualization and design, with input from the remaining authors. S. O. Bell and A. Gemmill secured the funding. All authors were involved in data acquisition, analysis, and interpretation, though A. M. Franks led the analysis. S. O. Bell, A. M. Franks, A. Feller, and A. Gemmill led the drafting of the article while the remaining authors provided critical review. All authors approved the final version of the article for publication. S. O. Bell, A. M. Franks, A. Feller, and A. Gemmill had full access to all of the data in the study and take responsibility for the integrity of the data and the accuracy of the analysis.

ACKNOWLEDGMENTS

This study was supported by grants P2CHD042854 and R01HD114292 from the National Institute of Child Health and Human Development.

We thank Marie Thoma and Blair Berger for their invaluable input on this article.

CONFLICTS OF INTEREST

The authors have no conflicts of interest to disclose.

HUMAN PARTICIPATION PROTECTION

The Johns Hopkins Bloomberg School of Public Health institutional review board provided ethical approval for this study (No. 29587).

REFERENCES

1. *New York Times*. Tracking the states where abortion is banned. April 3, 2025. Available at: https://www.nytimes.com/interactive/2024/us/abortion-laws-roe-v-wade.html. Accessed February 19, 2026.
2. Aiken AR, Starling JE, Scott JG, Gomperts R. Requests for self-managed medication abortion provided using online telemedicine in 30 US states before and after the *Dobbs v Jackson Women's Health Organization* decision. *JAMA*. 2022;328(17):1768–1770. https://doi.org/10.1001/jama.2022.18865
3. Society of Family Planning, Upadhyay U, Norris A. #WeCount report April 2022 through June 2024. 2024.
4. Maddow-Zimet I, Philbin J, DoCampo I, Jones RK, Monthly Abortion Provision Study, Updated March 24, 2026. Available at: https://osf.io/k4x7t. Accessed April 8, 2026.

5. Bell SO, Stuart EA, Gemmill A. Texas' 2021 ban on abortion in early pregnancy and changes in live births. *JAMA.* 2023;330(3):281–282. https://doi.org/10.1001/jama.2023.12034
6. Bell SO, Franks AM, Arbour D, et al. US abortion bans and fertility. *JAMA.* 2025;333(15):1324–1332. https://doi.org/10.1001/jama.2024.28527
7. Myers CK, Dench DL, Pineda-Torres M. The road not taken: how driving distance and appointment availability shape the effects of abortion bans. National Bureau of Economic Research. 2025. NBER working paper 33548. https://doi.org/10.3386/w33548
8. Caraher R. Do abortion bans affect reproductive and infant health? Evidence from Texas's 2021 ban and its impact on health disparities. July 30, 2024. Available at: https://papers.ssrn.com/abstract=4911886. Accessed August 26, 2024.
9. Gemmill A, Franks AM, Anjur-Dietrich S, et al. US abortion bans and infant mortality. *JAMA.* 2025;333(15):1315–1323. https://doi.org/10.1001/jama.2024.28517
10. Gemmill A, Margerison CE, Stuart EA, Bell SO. Infant deaths after Texas' 2021 ban on abortion in early pregnancy. *JAMA Pediatr.* 2024;178(8): 784–791. https://doi.org/10.1001/jamapediatrics.2024.0885
11. Hoyert DL. Maternal mortality rates in the United States, 2023. National Center for Health Statistics. 2025. Available at: https://www.cdc.gov/nchs/data/hestat/maternal-mortality/2023/maternal-mortality-rates-2023.htm. Accessed April 4, 2025.
12. Gunja MZ, Gumas ED, Masitha R, Zephyrin LC. Insights into the US maternal mortality crisis: an international comparison. The Commonwealth Fund. June 4, 2024. Available at: https://www.commonwealthfund.org/publications/issue-briefs/2024/jun/insights-us-maternal-mortality-crisis-international-comparison. Accessed April 4, 2025.
13. Trost SL, Beauregard J, Petersen EE, et al. Identifying deaths during and after pregnancy: new approaches to a perennial challenge. *Public Health Rep.* 2023;138(4):567–572. https://doi.org/10.1177/00333549221110487
14. Centers for Disease Control and Prevention, National Center for Health Statistics. National Vital Statistics System, Mortality 2018-2023 on CDC WONDER Online Database. Released in 2024. Available at: https://www.google.com/url?q=http://wonder.cdc.gov/ucd-icd10-expanded.html&sa=D&source=docs&ust=1762709807231797&usg=AOvVaw1ntDjKNfNC7xBHo2g-kcEc. Accessed November 5, 2025.
15. Treder KM, Amutah-Onukagha N, White KO. Abortion bans will exacerbate already severe racial inequities in maternal mortality. *Womens Health Issues.* 2023;33(4):328–332. https://doi.org/10.1016/j.whi.2023.04.007
16. Kaiser Family Foundation. Policy tracker: exceptions to state abortion bans and early gestational limits. Available at: https://www.kff.org/womens-health-policy/dashboard/exceptions-in-state-abortion-bans-and-early-gestational-limits. Accessed April 4, 2025.
17. Raymond EG, Grimes DA. The comparative safety of legal induced abortion and childbirth in the United States. *Obstet Gynecol.* 2012;119(2 pt 1): 215–219. https://doi.org/10.1097/AOG.0b013e31823fe923
18. Steenland MW, Mercon K, Brown BP, Thoma ME. Pregnancy- and abortion-related mortality in the US, 2018–2021. *JAMA Netw Open.* 2026;9(1): e2554793–e2554793. https://doi.org/10.1001/jamanetworkopen.2025.54793
19. Margerison CE, Wang X, Goldman-Mellor S, Muzik M, Gemmill A. Changes in racial and ethnic inequities in pregnancy-associated death in the United States during the COVID-19 pandemic. *Am J Public Health.* 2024;114(7):733–742. https://doi.org/10.2105/AJPH.2024.307651
20. Thoma ME, Declercq ER. Changes in pregnancy-related mortality associated with the coronavirus disease 2019 (COVID-19) pandemic in the United States. *Obstet Gynecol.* 2023;141(5):911–917. https://doi.org/10.1097/AOG.0000000000005182
21. Stevenson AJ. The pregnancy-related mortality impact of a total abortion ban in the United States: a research note on increased deaths due to remaining pregnant. *Demography.* 2021;58(6): 2019–2028. https://doi.org/10.1215/00703370-9585908
22. Henry NJ, Bintz C, Arndt MB, et al. Access to abortion and maternal health in a post-Roe world: a simulation study. Paper presented at: Population Association of America Annual Meeting; New Orleans, LA; April 12–15, 2023.
23. ProPublica. Life of the mother: how abortion bans lead to preventable deaths. Available at: https://www.propublica.org/series/life-of-the-mother. Accessed April 4, 2025.
24. Hoyert DL, Uddin SFG, Minino AM. *Evaluation of the Pregnancy Status Checkbox on the Identification of Maternal Deaths*. Hyattsville, MD: National Center for Health Statistics; 2020.
25. Ahmed SMA, Cresswell JA, Say L. Incompleteness and misclassification of maternal death recording: a systematic review and meta-analysis. *BMC Pregnancy Childbirth.* 2023;23(1):794. https://doi.org/10.1186/s12884-023-06077-4
26. Peterson E, Chou D, Moller AB, Gemmill A, Say L, Alkema L. Estimating misclassification errors in the reporting of maternal mortality in national civil registration vital statistics systems: a Bayesian hierarchical bivariate random walk model to estimate sensitivity and specificity for multiple countries and years with missing data. *Stat Med.* 2022;41(14): 2483–2496. https://doi.org/10.1002/sim.9335
27. Catalano A, Davis NL, Petersen EE, et al. Pregnant? Validity of the pregnancy checkbox on death certificates in four states, and characteristics associated with pregnancy checkbox errors. *Am J Obstet Gynecol.* 2020;222(3):269.e1–269.e8. https://doi.org/10.1016/j.ajog.2019.10.005
28. Baeva S, Saxton DL, Ruggiero K, et al. Identifying maternal deaths in Texas using an enhanced method, 2012. *Obstet Gynecol.* 2018;131(5): 762–769. https://doi.org/10.1097/AOG.0000000000002565
29. Hoyert DL. Maternal mortality rates in the United States, 2021. National Center for Health Statistics. 2023. Available at: https://www.cdc.gov/nchs/data/hestat/maternal-mortality/2021/maternal-mortality-rates-2021.htm. Accessed April 4, 2025.
30. Rossen LM, Hoyert DL, Horon I, Branum AM. Trends in maternal mortality rates by state, United States, 2018 to 2023. *Am J Obstet Gynecol.* 2026;234(1):250–269. https://doi.org/10.1016/j.ajog.2025.08.028
31. National Center for Health Statistics. Restricted-use vital statistics data. 2024. Available at: https://www.cdc.gov/nchs/nvss/nvss-restricted-data.htm. Accessed April 4, 2025.
32. Margerison CE, Roberts MH, Gemmill A, Goldman-Mellor S. Pregnancy-associated deaths due to drugs, suicide, and homicide in the United States, 2010–2019. *Obstet Gynecol.* 2022;139(2):172–180. https://doi.org/10.1097/AOG.0000000000004649
33. Chen Y, Shiels MS, Uribe-Leitz T, et al. Pregnancy-related deaths in the US, 2018–2022. *JAMA Netw Open.* 2025;8(4):e254325. https://doi.org/10.1001/jamanetworkopen.2025.4325
34. Singh P, Crawford A, Crow S, Powell JR, Gallo MF. Suicide deaths among reproductive-aged women in the US post-Dobbs: a national time-series analysis. *Soc Psychiatry Psychiatr Epidemiol.* 2025; 60(8):1835–1845. https://doi.org/10.1007/s00127-025-02902-7
35. Declercq E, Barnard-Mayers R, Zephyrin L, Johnson K. The US maternal health divide: the limited maternal health services and worse outcomes of states proposing new abortion restrictions. The Commonwealth Fund. 2022. Available at: https://www.commonwealthfund.org/publications/issue-briefs/2022/dec/us-maternal-health-divide-limited-services-worse-outcomes. Accessed April 4, 2025.
36. Hill L, Artiga S, Ranji U, Gomez I, Ndugga N. What are the implications of the Dobbs ruling for racial disparities? KFF. April 24, 2024. Available at: https://www.kff.org/womens-health-policy/issue-brief/what-are-the-implications-of-the-dobbs-ruling-for-racial-disparities. Accessed June 13, 2025.
37. Hawkins SS, Baum CF. Severe maternal morbidity in the United States. Econofact. March 20, 2023. Available at: https://econofact.org/severe-maternal-morbidity-in-the-united-states. Accessed April 4, 2025.
38. Presser L, Suozzo A, Chou S, Surana K. Texas banned abortion. Then sepsis rates soared. ProPublica. February 20, 2025. Available at: https://www.propublica.org/article/texas-abortion-ban-sepsis-maternal-mortality-analysis. Accessed April 4, 2025.
39. Surana K, Presser L, Suozzo A. A "striking" trend: after Texas banned abortion, more women nearly bled to death during miscarriage. ProPublica. July 1, 2025. Available at: https://www.propublica.org/article/texas-abortion-ban-miscarriage-blood-transfusions. Accessed August 20, 2025.
40. Nagle A, Samari G, Thaxton L, Gemmill A. Blood transfusions for pregnancy loss in Texas before and after abortion bans, 2017–2023. *Am J Public Health.* 2025;115(11):1887–1894. https://doi.org/10.2105/AJPH.2025.308224
41. Ungar L. Maternal mortality review panels are in the spotlight. Here's what they do. AP News. December 5, 2024. Available at: https://apnews.com/article/maternal-mortality-cdc-abortion-georgia-texas-idaho-10dae96d52503709f4beb698a3f12db5. Accessed April 4, 2025.
42. Austin N, Harper S. Constructing a longitudinal database of targeted regulation of abortion providers laws. *Health Serv Res.* 2019;54(5):1084–1089. https://doi.org/10.1111/1475-6773.13185
43. Callahan T, Zaharatos J, St Pierre A, Merkt PT, Goodman D. Enhancing reviews and surveillance to eliminate maternal mortality. *J Womens Health (Larchmt).* 2021;30(8):1068–1073. https://doi.org/10.1089/jwh.2021.0357
44. Collier ARY, Molina RL. Maternal mortality in the United States: updates on trends, causes, and solutions. *Neoreviews.* 2019;20(10):e561–e574. https://doi.org/10.1542/neo.20-10-e561

Racial/Ethnic Differences in Homicides of Adult Women and the Role of Intimate Partner Violence: United States, 2018–2022

Kaitlin Forsberg, MPH, Katherine A. Fowler, PhD, Bridget H. Lyons, MPH, Shane P. D. Jack, PhD, and Janet M. Blair, PhD, MPH

Objectives. To describe rates and characteristics of homicides of women across racial/ethnic groups, and describe intimate partner violence (IPV)–related and non–IPV-related homicide circumstances across racial/ethnic groups.

Methods. We used National Vital Statistics System data to calculate homicide rates by racial/ethnic group of US women (aged ≥ 18 years) who were homicide victims from 2018 to 2022. We used National Violent Death Reporting System data to characterize the circumstances and suspects in these homicides by racial/ethnic group and IPV involvement.

Results. The age-adjusted homicide rate was 3.2 per 100 000 women. Rates for non-Hispanic Black women and non-Hispanic American Indian/Alaska Native women were more than twice as high as those for other races/ethnicities. Most women were killed by a firearm (67.9%), fatally injured in a residence (64.8%), or killed by a male (92.5%). About half (47.3%) of homicides were IPV related. Non–IPV-related homicides were often perpetrated by family members (39.0%). Circumstances differed by racial/ethnic group.

Conclusions. Homicide disproportionally affects certain racial/ethnic groups of women, and the characteristics of homicides differ across groups. Thorough examination of these differences could aid in effective, targeted homicide prevention. (*Am J Public Health*. 2026;116(6):829–840. https://doi.org/10.2105/AJPH.2026.308461)

AJPH June 2026, Vol. 116, No. 6

Violence against women is an urgent public health issue.[1] US women are less likely to die violently than are US men, yet thousands each year are victims of homicide, and the consequences of these deaths are far-reaching. In the United States in 2023, more than 4500 girls and women died by homicide.[2] Although homicides can occur among women of all ages and backgrounds, the risk of homicide varies by age, pregnancy status, and race/ethnicity.[3–5]

Intimate partner violence (IPV) is frequently associated with these homicides.[6–8] An analysis of 2022 national data on violent deaths found that in 51% of homicides of females in which the relationship between the perpetrator and victim was known, the victim was killed by a current or former intimate partner.[8] Even that does not convey the full extent of IPV-related homicides, as a substantial proportion of victims in such incidents are corollary victims (i.e., family, friends, neighbors, and persons who intervene, including law enforcement or bystanders), not intimate partners.[7,9,10]

In 2017, Petrosky et al. conducted an analysis of racial/ethnic differences in homicides of women using 2003–2014 National Violent Death Reporting System (NVDRS) data.[11] They found that homicide rates among non-Hispanic Black and non-Hispanic American Indian/Alaska Native (AIAN) women were more than 2 times that of Hispanic, non-Hispanic White, and non-Hispanic Asian/Pacific Islander women as well as that half of homicides of women were IPV related. An update of this work is needed. Recent analyses show that homicides of women have increased in recent years, particularly during the COVID-19 pandemic.[5] Additionally, NVDRS has expanded jurisdictional participation and data elements since the Petrosky et al. analysis, providing a more comprehensive picture. Finally, the US Census Bureau revised its population data reporting, transitioning to single-race population estimates.[12] This change ensures that people who identify as more than 1 race—including multiracial women—are fully counted.[12]

In our analysis, we characterized homicides of women across racial/ethnic groups to better understand the circumstances and context surrounding these incidents and to inform prevention. We had 2 objectives: (1) to describe the frequency of demographic and fatal injury characteristics of homicides of women, comparing decedents across racial/ethnic groups, and (2) to describe the role of IPV in these homicides and the circumstances related to homicides with and without IPV across racial/ethnic groups.

METHODS

We conducted a cross-sectional analysis of US women (aged ≥ 18 years) who were homicide victims between 2018 and 2022 (the most recent years that single-race population or case data were available at the time of our analysis).[4,8,12]

Data Sources

We used 2 data sources: the National Vital Statistics System (NVSS) and NVDRS.[13] NVDRS includes detailed information about homicide victims, suspects, injuries, and circumstances (including the role of IPV) but is not yet nationally representative[8] and therefore could not be used to calculate national homicide rates. To calculate homicide rates, we used NVSS data, which accounts for all homicides in the 50 US states and the District of Columbia during the study period.

National Vital Statistics System. We examined homicide rates by race/ethnicity using the NVSS (death certificate) data from all 50 states and the District of Columbia via the US Centers for Disease Control and Prevention's (CDC's) web-based Injury Statistics Query and Reporting System.[4] Cases included all homicides of women aged 18 years and older between 2018 and 2022.

National Violent Death Reporting System. NVDRS is a public health surveillance system that collects data on violent deaths and suicides, including homicides. NVDRS has been described in detail previously.[8] Data collection is coordinated at the state or jurisdictional level and comprises 3 primary data sources: death certificates, coroner and medical examiner reports, and law enforcement reports. NVDRS collects a range of variables, including victim and suspected perpetrator (hereafter "suspect") demographic information, characteristics of the injuries, and precipitating circumstances surrounding the death.

We included NVDRS homicide cases from all 50 US states, the District of Columbia, and Puerto Rico for 2018 to 2022; yearly participation was subject to funding and data quality (Table A, available as a supplement to the online version of this article at http://www.ajph.org). We included homicide victims if the victim's sex was female and age at death was 18 years or older. We excluded NVDRS cases if age or sex were unknown or race/ethnicity was unknown or "other."

NVDRS is uniquely suited for IPV-related homicide analyses, as it includes the relationship between the homicide victim and the homicide suspect and has an "intimate partner violence–related" circumstance variable indicating that the death was related to a conflict or violence between current or former intimate partners. Similar to the study of Petrosky et al.,[11] we considered incidents IPV related if a homicide or legal intervention death (i.e., death caused by law enforcement and other persons with legal authority to use deadly force acting in the line of duty) in the incident was marked as "intimate partner violence related" or if a person killed their current or former intimate partner. We also considered deaths of corollary victims (i.e., victims killed owing to intimate partner–related conflict/violence who were not the intimate partner) IPV related.

Analysis

For the NVSS analysis, we generated age-adjusted homicide rates using the National Center for Health Statistics 2000 US standard population.[14] For the NVDRS analysis, we conducted descriptive analyses to assess victim demographics and homicide characteristics across race/ethnicity in SAS version 9.4 (SAS Institute, Cary, NC). We examined precipitating circumstances and suspect characteristics across race/ethnicity separately for IPV-related deaths and non–IPV-related deaths. We used the χ^2 test to compare race/ethnicity groups. We considered a 2-sided *P* value of less than .05 significant. For each characteristic with statistically significant differences, we used post hoc pairwise comparisons using

AJPH June 2026, Vol. 116, No. 6

the χ^2 test with the Bonferroni correction for multiple comparisons to determine which of the 6 race/ethnicity groups were significantly different from each other (15 pairwise comparisons using PROC MULTTEST in SAS to generate adjusted *P* values, which we assessed at < .05).

RESULTS

We first present our results from analyzing NVSS data describing homicide rates by race/ethnicity among US women and then our findings from NVDRS data describing victim characteristics, homicide circumstances, and suspect information, including analyses stratified by IPV involvement.

National Vital Statistics System

In the United States between 2018 and 2022, 19 709 women died by homicide (age-adjusted homicide rate = 3.2 per 100 000 women; Table 1). Non-Hispanic Black or African American (hereafter "non-Hispanic Black") women had the highest age-adjusted rate per 100 000 women (9.0), followed by non-Hispanic AIAN women (7.2), Hispanic or Latina (hereafter "Hispanic") women of any race (2.6), non-Hispanic women of 2 or more races (2.2), non-Hispanic White women (2.2), and non-Hispanic Asian, Native Hawaiian, or other Pacific Islander (ANHPI) women (1.1).

National Violent Death Reporting System

From 2018 to 2022, 16 081 homicides of women (Table 2) were reported in NVDRS, spanning 15 659 incidents (data not shown). Most incidents (75.8%) were single homicide events, and the rest (24.2%) involved multiple violent deaths, most commonly a homicide followed by a suicide (11.8% of incidents; data not shown).

By race/ethnicity, 6788 (42.2%) victims were non-Hispanic White, 6170 (38.4%) were non-Hispanic Black, 2262 (14.1%) were Hispanic, 363 (2.3%) were non-Hispanic ANHPI, 291 (1.8%) were non-Hispanic AIAN, and 207 (1.3%) were non-Hispanic women of 2 or more races. Approximately one quarter of victims (25.7%) were aged 25 to 34 years. Non-Hispanic White and non-Hispanic ANHPI victims were generally older than were victims from other racial/ethnic groups. More than 40% (44.6%) of victims were high school graduates or had a general equivalency diploma equivalent. Non-Hispanic AIAN and Hispanic victims generally had less education than did other racial/ethnic groups. Half of victims (50.8%) were never married or were single; this was highest among non-Hispanic Black victims. When pregnancy status was known (n = 3216), we found that approximately 13.8% of women of reproductive age (18–44 years) were pregnant or 6 or less weeks postpartum, including about a third (31.0%) of victims who were non-Hispanic women of 2 or more races and a quarter (26.8%) of non-Hispanic ANHPI victims. More than three quarters of victims were in the workforce.[15] A small proportion of victims (1.3%; data not shown) were noted to be lesbian, bisexual, or another sexual minority.

Firearms were used in more than two thirds (67.9%) of homicides, most frequently against non-Hispanic Black victims (78.6%). Homicides occurred most frequently in large central metro areas (37.9%) based on the 2013 National Center for Health Statistics urban–rural classification scheme for counties,[16] but this differed significantly by race/ethnicity. Nearly half (48.1%) of homicides of non-Hispanic AIAN women occurred in nonmetropolitan (i.e., micropolitan or noncore) areas.[16] Most homicides took

TABLE 1— Number and Rates of Homicides of Women Aged ≥ 18 Years by Victim Race/Ethnicity: National Vital Statistics System, 50 US States and District of Columbia, 2018–2022

Race/Ethnicity	No. of Women Who Died by Homicide	Age-Adjusted Rate per 100 000 Women
Non-Hispanic Black/African American	7 268	9.0
Non-Hispanic American Indian/Alaska Native	323	7.2
Hispanic	2 878	2.6
Non-Hispanic ≥ 2 races	269	2.2
Non-Hispanic White	8 448	2.2
Non-Hispanic Asian/Native Hawaiian/Pacific Islander	483	1.1
Unknown	40	
Total	19 709	3.2

TABLE 2— Victim and Fatal Injury Characteristics of Homicides of Women Aged ≥18 Years by Victim Race/Ethnicity: National Violent Death Reporting System, 50 US States, District of Columbia, and Puerto Rico, 2018–2022

Characteristic	Total (n = 16 081), No. (%)	Non-Hispanic White (n = 6 788), No. (%)	Non-Hispanic Black/African American (n = 6 170), No. (%)	Non-Hispanic ANHPI (n = 363), No. (%)	Non-Hispanic AIAN (n = 291), No. (%)	Non-Hispanic ≥2 Races (n = 207), No. (%)	Hispanic (n = 2 262), No. (%)
Age, y							
18–24	2 794 (17.4)	643 (9.5)	1 471 (23.8)	30 (8.3)	52 (17.9)	61 (29.5)	537 (23.7)
25–34	4 134 (25.7)	1 304 (19.2)	1 940 (31.4)	70 (19.3)	81 (27.8)	63 (30.4)	676 (29.9)
35–44	3 196 (19.9)	1 336 (19.7)	1 196 (19.4)	73 (20.1)	71 (24.4)	37 (17.9)	483 (21.4)
45–54	2 247 (14.0)	1 093 (16.1)	722 (11.7)	68 (18.7)	40 (13.7)	24 (11.6)	300 (13.3)
55–64	1 722 (10.7)	1 003 (14.8)	490 (7.9)	51 (14.0)	23 (7.9)	9 (4.3)	146 (6.5)
≥65	1 988 (12.4)	1 409 (20.8)	351 (5.7)	71 (19.6)	24 (8.2)	13 (6.3)	120 (5.3)
Education (among those with known education; n = 15 756)							
<High school graduate or GED equivalent	3 021 (19.2)	1 059 (15.9)	1 091 (18.0)	51 (14.5)	89 (31.3)	28 (13.8)	703 (31.9)
High school graduate or GED equivalent	7 030 (44.6)	2 903 (43.7)	2 958 (48.8)	109 (31.1)	103 (36.3)	89 (43.8)	868 (39.4)
Some college or more	5 705 (36.2)	2 685 (40.4)	2 017 (33.3)	191 (54.4)	92 (32.4)	86 (42.4)	634 (28.8)
Marital status (among those with known status; n = 15 893)							
Married, civil union, or domestic partnership	3 834 (24.1)	2 246 (33.5)	824 (13.5)	151 (42.2)	50 (17.4)	42 (20.4)	521 (23.4)
Never married or single	8 066 (50.8)	2 017 (30.1)	4 405 (72.1)	86 (24.0)	160 (55.6)	130 (63.1)	1 268 (56.9)
Separated, divorced, or widowed	3 993 (25.1)	2 442 (36.4)	879 (14.4)	121 (33.8)	78 (27.1)	34 (16.5)	439 (19.7)
Pregnant or ≤6 wk postpartum (those aged 18–44 y with known status; n = 3216)	445 (13.8)	99 (9.0)	233 (16.1)	11 (26.8)	9 (15.5)	13 (31.0)	80 (15.2)
Usual occupation[a] (those with known occupation; n = 13 938)							
In workforce	11 073 (79.4)	4 717 (77.3)	4 331 (83.8)	257 (79.1)	184 (71.0)	138 (76.7)	1 446 (75.9)
Not in workforce	2 865 (20.6)	1 383 (22.7)	838 (16.2)	68 (20.9)	75 (29.0)	42 (23.3)	459 (24.1)
Methods of injury (among those with known method; n = 15 382)							
Firearm	10 445 (67.9)	3 880 (59.9)	4 730 (78.6)	184 (54.8)	141 (52.2)	134 (70.2)	1 376 (65.9)
Sharp instrument	2 390 (15.5)	1 112 (17.2)	728 (12.1)	74 (22.0)	63 (23.3)	22 (11.5)	391 (18.7)
Blunt instrument	1 078 (7.0)	651 (10.1)	216 (3.6)	32 (9.5)	28 (10.4)	9 (4.7)	142 (6.8)
Hanging, strangulation, suffocation	927 (6.0)	513 (7.9)	230 (3.8)	26 (7.7)	13 (4.8)	12 (6.3)	133 (6.4)
Personal weapons	565 (3.7)	332 (5.1)	107 (1.8)	21 (6.3)	29 (10.7)	11 (5.8)	65 (3.1)
Urban–rural injury location[b] (among those with known location; n = 15 514)							
Large central metro	5 886 (37.9)	1 479 (22.4)	3 106 (51.3)	186 (51.8)	38 (13.4)	63 (31.8)	1 014 (50.3)
Large fringe metro	2 604 (16.8)	1 256 (19.0)	913 (15.1)	74 (20.6)	20 (7.1)	37 (18.7)	304 (15.1)
Medium metro	3 316 (21.4)	1 589 (24.1)	1 118 (18.5)	64 (17.8)	55 (19.4)	50 (25.3)	440 (21.8)

Continued

TABLE 2— Continued

Characteristic	Total (n = 16 081), No. (%)	Non-Hispanic White (n = 6 788), No. (%)	Non-Hispanic Black/African American (n = 6 170), No. (%)	Non-Hispanic ANHPI (n = 363), No. (%)	Non-Hispanic AIAN (n = 291), No. (%)	Non-Hispanic ≥2 Races (n = 207), No. (%)	Hispanic (n = 2 262), No. (%)
Small metro	1 440 (9.3)	837 (12.7)	423 (7.0)	18 (5.0)	34 (12.0)	16 (8.1)	112 (5.6)
Micropolitan (nonmetropolitan)	1 324 (8.5)	806 (12.2)	305 (5.0)	7 (1.9)	82 (29.0)	19 (9.6)	105 (5.2)
Noncore (nonmetropolitan)	944 (6.1)	638 (9.7)	189 (3.1)	10 (2.8)	54 (19.1)	13 (6.6)	40 (2.0)
Type of injury location (among those with known location; n = 15 017)							
House/apartment	9 736 (64.8)	4 731 (74.4)	3 281 (56.4)	220 (67.3)	182 (66.7)	114 (62.6)	1 208 (58.5)
Street/road, sidewalk, alley	1 572 (10.5)	345 (5.4)	902 (15.5)	21 (6.4)	20 (7.3)	23 (12.6)	261 (12.6)
Motor vehicle (excluding school bus and public transportation)	1 516 (10.1)	363 (5.7)	838 (14.4)	16 (4.9)	18 (6.6)	13 (7.1)	268 (13.0)
Other	2 193 (14.6)	916 (14.4)	795 (13.7)	70 (21.4)	53 (19.4)	32 (17.6)	327 (15.8)
Victim injured at own home (among those with known home location status; n = 14 406)	7 562 (52.5)	3 876 (63.8)	2 351 (41.8)	193 (60.7)	128 (48.9)	82 (44.8)	932 (47.9)

Note. ANHPI = Asian, Native Hawaiian, or other Pacific Islander; AIAN = American Indian or Alaska Native; GED = general equivalency diploma. We assessed pairwise racial/ethnic comparisons using the Bonferroni-corrected χ^2 test; all characteristics differed significantly across racial/ethnic groups ($P < .05$).

[a]Usual occupation participation in the workforce was based on the National Institute for Occupational Safety and Health Industry and Occupation Computerized Coding System output to the 2018 Standard Occupational Classification system.[15]

[b]The urban–rural designations of injury location county are based on the 2013 National Center for Health Statistics urban–rural classification scheme for counties, which does not include Puerto Rico.[16]

place at a house or apartment (64.8%). In more than half of homicides (52.5%), the victim was fatally injured at her own home.

IPV-related homicides of women. Because IPV is considered a circumstance precipitating homicide in NVDRS, we included only cases with circumstance data available in analyses examining IPV-related and non–IPV-related homicides. Therefore, circumstances were known for all IPV-related homicides (n = 5916); 6581 (64.7%) of the remaining homicides had circumstance information and therefore made up the non–IPV-related group. Nearly half (49.1%) of the IPV-related homicides were of non-Hispanic White women, followed by victims who were non-Hispanic Black (29.8%), Hispanic (15.3%), non-Hispanic ANHPI (2.8%), non-Hispanic AIAN (1.7%), and non-Hispanic women of 2 or more races (1.4%; Table 3). In 41.5% of IPV-related cases, an argument or conflict preceded the death, most commonly among non-Hispanic Black and non-Hispanic AIAN victims.

The victim–suspect relationship was known for 5528 IPV-related homicides. Of these, 4383 (79.3%) were perpetrated by a current intimate partner, 816 (14.8%) were perpetrated by a former intimate partner, and 329 (6.0%) were perpetrated by someone other than an intimate partner. Nearly all suspects were male (97.4% of homicides in which suspect's sex was known; data not shown). About half of suspects with a known age were aged 25 to 44 years, and two thirds of IPV-related homicides in which the suspect's race/ethnicity was known were perpetrated by suspects with the same race/ethnicity as the victim.

TABLE 3— Circumstances and Suspect Characteristics of Intimate Partner Violence–Related Homicides of Women Aged ≥ 18 Years by Victim Race/Ethnicity: National Violent Death Reporting System, 50 US States, District of Columbia, and Puerto Rico, 2018–2022

Characteristic	Total (n = 5 916), No. (%)	Non-Hispanic White (n = 2 903), No. (%)	Non-Hispanic Black/African American (n = 1 763), No. (%)	Non-Hispanic ANHPI (n = 168), No. (%)	Non-Hispanic AIAN (n = 98), No. (%)	Non-Hispanic ≥ 2 Races (n = 81), No. (%)	Hispanic (n = 903), No. (%)	P
Circumstances								
Argument or conflict preceded victim's death	2457 (41.5)	1 087 (37.4)	853 (48.4)	47 (28.0)	47 (48.0)	32 (39.5)	391 (43.3)	< .01
Victim experienced violence in the past month	515 (8.7)	290 (10.0)	131 (7.4)	11 (6.5)	11 (11.2)	5 (6.2)	67 (7.4)	.02
Jealousy/lovers' triangle	460 (7.8)	225 (7.8)	113 (6.4)	15 (8.9)	7 (7.1)	6 (7.4)	94 (10.4)	.02
Suspect characteristics[a]								
Victim–suspect relationship (among those with known relationship; n = 5528)								< .01
Current intimate partner	4 383 (79.3)	2 226 (82.1)	1 253 (76.1)	128 (81.5)	79 (84.9)	52 (68.4)	645 (76.2)	
Former intimate partner	816 (14.8)	320 (11.8)	288 (17.5)	23 (14.6)	10 (10.8)	14 (18.4)	161 (19.0)	
Other	329 (6.0)	164 (6.1)	105 (6.4)	6 (3.8)	4 (4.3)	10 (13.2)	40 (4.7)	
Age group of suspect, y (among those with known age; n = 4847)								< .01
< 18	11 (0.2)	2 (0.1)	8 (0.6)	0 (0)	0 (0)	0 (0)	1 (0.1)	
18–24	483 (10.0)	158 (6.3)	219 (15.7)	6 (4.3)	12 (19.7)	10 (15.2)	78 (11.5)	
25–34	1157 (23.9)	458 (18.3)	431 (30.8)	26 (18.4)	15 (24.6)	24 (36.4)	203 (30.0)	
35–44	1180 (24.3)	544 (21.7)	377 (26.9)	29 (20.6)	18 (29.5)	15 (22.7)	197 (29.1)	
45–54	872 (18.0)	491 (19.6)	202 (14.4)	33 (23.4)	10 (16.4)	9 (13.6)	127 (18.8)	
55–64	588 (12.1)	396 (15.8)	110 (7.9)	25 (17.7)	0 (0)	5 (7.6)	52 (7.7)	
≥ 65	556 (11.5)	454 (18.1)	52 (3.7)	22 (15.6)	6 (9.8)	3 (4.5)	19 (2.8)	
Race/ethnicity of suspect (among those with known race/ethnicity; n = 5430)								< .01
Different race/ethnicity than victim	1664 (30.6)	756 (28.4)	311 (19.0)	73 (47.7)	65 (74.7)	70 (95.9)	389 (47.7)	
Same race/ethnicity as victim	3766 (69.4)	1 906 (71.6)	1 329 (81.0)	80 (52.3)	22 (25.3)	3 (4.1)	426 (52.3)	
Suspect injury circumstances								
Suspect attempted or died by suicide after (n = 5767)	2 146 (37.2)	1 301 (45.7)	369 (21.6)	88 (53.7)	24 (25.5)	32 (41.0)	332 (37.9)	< .01
History of abuse of victim by suspect (n = 5742)	1049 (18.3)	500 (17.7)	292 (17.1)	27 (16.9)	31 (33.0)	12 (15.4)	187 (21.5)	< .01
Suspect had contact with law enforcement in past 12 mo (n = 5742)	830 (14.5)	427 (15.1)	220 (12.9)	17 (10.6)	22 (23.4)	22 (28.2)	122 (14.0)	< .01
Suspected alcohol use by suspect (n = 5742)	579 (10.1)	356 (12.6)	82 (4.8)	14 (8.8)	32 (34.0)	11 (14.1)	84 (9.7)	< .01
Suspected substance use (other than alcohol) by the suspect (n = 5742)	428 (7.5)	250 (8.8)	85 (5.0)	9 (5.6)	15 (16.0)	11 (14.1)	58 (6.7)	< .01

Note. ANHPI = Asian, Native Hawaiian, or other Pacific Islander; AIAN = American Indian or Alaska Native. We assessed racial/ethnic differences using the Bonferroni-corrected χ^2 test.
[a]Each death may have multiple suspects. However, to implement examination of suspect characteristics, we included only the primary suspect unless a different suspect was an intimate partner. If an intimate partner was listed as a suspect, we included that suspect to ensure proper intimate partner violence–related incident classification.

In 37.2% of IPV-related homicides, the suspect attempted or died by suicide after committing the homicide, including more than half of homicides of non-Hispanic ANHPI women and nearly half of homicides of non-Hispanic White women. A history of abuse by the suspect was known in 18.3% of IPV-related homicides, most commonly for non-Hispanic AIAN women (33.0%). The suspect had previous contact with law enforcement in 14.5% of homicides, most commonly for non-Hispanic women of 2 or more races (28.2%). The suspect was suspected of using alcohol in the hours preceding the incident in 10.1% of IPV-related homicides, most frequently among non-Hispanic AIAN women (34.0%).

Non–IPV-related homicides of women. Non-Hispanic Black women made up the largest proportion of the 6581 non–IPV-related homicides (43.0%) followed by victims who were non-Hispanic White (38.7%), Hispanic (13.0%), non-Hispanic AIAN (2.0%), non-Hispanic ANHPI (1.9%), and non-Hispanic women of 2 or more races (1.3%; Table 4).

Non–IPV-related homicides were most often precipitated by an argument or conflict (25.8%) or another crime (25.5%; most frequently assault/homicide [46.1%], robbery [25.5%], or burglary [12.3%]). Other commonly reported circumstances differed by race/ethnicity. For non-Hispanic White and non-Hispanic ANHPI victims, a family relationship problem was common (21.0% and 19.8%, respectively). For non-Hispanic Black victims, a frequent circumstance was a drive-by shooting (18.7%). For non-Hispanic AIAN victims, a physical fight between 2 people (18.9%), a family relationship problem (14.4%), or a problem with a friend or associate (14.4%) frequently preceded the homicide. A problem with a friend or associate was also common for victims of non-Hispanic women of 2 or more races (13.8%). For Hispanic victims, non–IPV-related homicides were often gang related (15.5%) or involved a drive-by shooting (15.4%).

The victim–suspect relationship was known for 3167 non–IPV-related homicides. Among those, the victim's relationship to the suspect was parent (21.2%), stranger (18.1%), other family member (17.7%), acquaintance (14.1%), or other relationship (28.9%). The most common relationships by race/ethnicity were as follows: non-Hispanic ANHPI victims were parents of the suspect (30.3%), non-Hispanic AIAN victims were other family members (29.2%), and non-Hispanic victims of 2 or more races were strangers (25.0%); for all other racial/ethnic groups, the most common relationship group was "other" (non-Hispanic Black = 31.0%; Hispanic = 29.5%; non-Hispanic White = 28.4%).

Most non–IPV-related homicides in which suspect sex was known had male suspects (86.3%; data not shown). In nearly a third of non–IPV-related homicides with known suspect ages, the suspect was aged 25 to 34 years. In about half of non–IPV-related homicides with known suspect race/ethnicity, the suspect was the same race/ethnicity as the victim (52.7%) although this ranged significantly from 2.9% for non-Hispanic victims of 2 or more races to 62.3% for non-Hispanic Black victims.

The suspect had previous law enforcement contact in 11.3% of non–IPV-related homicides and was reported more frequently in homicides involving non-Hispanic victims of 2 or more races (21.1%) or non-Hispanic White victims (14.9%) than homicides of Hispanic (8.5%) or non-Hispanic Black (8.1%) victims. The homicide was directly attributed to the suspect's mental illness in 8.2% of non–IPV-related homicides overall, with the highest percentages for non-Hispanic ANHPI (13.3%) and non-Hispanic White (12.9%) victim homicides. Suspects were suspected of substance use (other than alcohol) in 17.1% of homicides of non-Hispanic victims of 2 or more races. In 6.0% of non–IPV-related homicides, the suspect attempted or died by suicide, and, in non-Hispanic ANHPI homicides, 16.8% of suspects attempted or died by suicide.

DISCUSSION

We examined the frequency and characteristics of homicides of women in the United States, finding a homicide rate for adult women that was 60% higher than the rate of 2.0 per 100 000 women found in the analysis of Petrosky et al. of 2003 to 2014 data.[11] Unlike the Petrosky et al. analysis, our investigation covered the time during the COVID-19 pandemic and included a separate category for non-Hispanic women of 2 or more races; for the NVDRS analysis, our study included a wider range of jurisdictions. We found that homicide rates were 4.1 times higher among non-Hispanic Black women and 3.3 times higher among non-Hispanic AIAN women than among non-Hispanic White women, mirroring previous studies.[5,8]

When compared with the results of Petrosky et al., our results had a higher proportion of firearm homicides (67.9% vs 53.4%).[11] We also found a greater proportion of women who were never married or were single compared with the previous study (50.8% vs 38.2%). Among the IPV-related homicides, we found a higher proportion preceded by

TABLE 4— Circumstances and Suspect Characteristics of Non-Intimate Partner Violence–Related Homicides of Women Aged ≥ 18 Years by Victim Race/Ethnicity: National Violent Death Reporting System, 50 US States, District of Columbia, and Puerto Rico, 2018–2022

Characteristic	Total (n = 6 581), No. (%)	Non-Hispanic White (n = 2 546), No. (%)	Non-Hispanic Black or African American (n = 2 833), No. (%)	Non-Hispanic ANHPI (n = 126), No. (%)	Non-Hispanic AIAN (n = 132), No. (%)	Non-Hispanic ≥2 Races (n = 87), No. (%)	Hispanic (n = 857), No. (%)	P
Circumstances								
Argument or conflict preceded victim's death	1 696 (25.8)	619 (24.3)	779 (27.5)	26 (20.6)	36 (27.3)	27 (31.0)	209 (24.4)	.05
Precipitated by another crime	1 681 (25.5)	751 (29.5)	644 (22.7)	51 (40.5)	32 (24.2)	21 (24.1)	182 (21.2)	< .01
Assault or homicide	775 (46.1)	308 (41.0)	349 (54.2)	29 (56.9)	10 (31.3)	13 (61.9)	66 (36.3)	
Robbery	428 (25.5)	206 (27.4)	139 (21.6)	20 (39.2)	7 (21.9)	4 (19.1)	52 (28.6)	
Burglary	206 (12.3)	111 (14.8)	69 (10.7)	7 (13.7)	2 (6.3)	2 (9.5)	15 (8.2)	
Relationship problem with a family member (other than an intimate partner)	936 (14.2)	535 (21.0)	255 (9.0)	25 (19.8)	19 (14.4)	11 (12.6)	91 (10.6)	< .01
Drive-by shooting	757 (11.5)	78 (3.1)	530 (18.7)	5 (4.0)	6 (4.5)	6 (6.9)	132 (15.4)	< .01
Physical fight between 2 people	601 (9.1)	226 (8.9)	255 (9.0)	13 (10.3)	25 (18.9)	9 (10.3)	73 (8.5)	.01
Drug involvement	597 (9.1)	257 (10.1)	213 (7.5)	9 (7.1)	10 (7.6)	8 (9.2)	100 (11.7)	< .01
Problem with a friend or associate (other than an intimate partner or family member)	509 (7.7)	240 (9.4)	149 (5.3)	5 (4.0)	19 (14.4)	12 (13.8)	84 (9.8)	< .01
Victim was a bystander	458 (7.0)	86 (3.4)	267 (9.4)	4 (3.2)	2 (1.5)	6 (6.9)	93 (10.9)	< .01
Gang related	360 (5.5)	49 (1.9)	167 (5.9)	1 (0.8)	6 (4.6)	4 (4.6)	133 (15.5)	< .01
Suspect characteristics[a]								
Victim–suspect relationship (among those with known relationship; n = 3167)								< .01
Parent	672 (21.2)	429 (27.0)	140 (13.8)	23 (30.3)	8 (11.1)	6 (11.5)	66 (18.0)	
Stranger	573 (18.1)	231 (14.5)	207 (20.5)	17 (22.4)	12 (16.7)	13 (25.0)	93 (25.4)	
Other family	560 (17.7)	284 (17.9)	172 (17.0)	14 (18.4)	21 (29.2)	11 (21.2)	58 (15.8)	
Acquaintance	446 (14.1)	195 (12.3)	179 (17.7)	3 (3.9)	17 (23.6)	11 (21.2)	41 (11.2)	
Other	916 (28.9)	451 (28.4)	313 (31.0)	19 (25.0)	14 (19.4)	11 (21.2)	108 (29.5)	
Age group of suspect, y (among those with known age; n = 3434)								< .01
< 18	172 (5.0)	68 (4.1)	65 (5.2)	4 (5.6)	2 (3.4)	3 (5.8)	30 (8.4)	
18–24	847 (24.7)	318 (19.4)	390 (31.1)	18 (25.4)	13 (22.0)	12 (23.1)	96 (27.0)	
25–34	1 096 (31.9)	471 (28.7)	436 (34.7)	21 (29.6)	21 (35.6)	23 (44.2)	124 (34.8)	
35–44	596 (17.4)	329 (20.0)	185 (14.7)	12 (16.9)	12 (20.3)	5 (9.6)	53 (14.9)	
45–54	356 (10.4)	214 (13.0)	98 (7.8)	7 (9.9)	4 (6.8)	6 (11.5)	27 (7.6)	
55–64	233 (6.8)	151 (9.2)	51 (4.1)	6 (8.5)	5 (8.5)	1 (1.9)	19 (5.3)	

Continued

TABLE 4— Continued

Characteristic	Total (n = 6 581), No. (%)	Non-Hispanic White (n = 2 546), No. (%)	Non-Hispanic Black or African American (n = 2 833), No. (%)	Non-Hispanic ANHPI (n = 126), No. (%)	Non-Hispanic AIAN (n = 132), No. (%)	Non-Hispanic ≥2 Races (n = 87), No. (%)	Hispanic (n = 857), No. (%)	*P*
≥65	134 (3.9)	90 (5.5)	30 (2.4)	3 (4.2)	2 (3.4)	2 (3.9)	7 (2.0)	
Race/ethnicity of suspect (among those with known race/ethnicity; n = 4944)								< .01
Different race/ethnicity than victim	2 340 (47.3)	963 (47.0)	760 (37.7)	76 (75.2)	85 (78.0)	67 (97.1)	389 (64.9)	
Same race/ethnicity as victim	2 604 (52.7)	1 085 (53.0)	1 258 (62.3)	25 (24.8)	24 (22.0)	2 (2.9)	210 (35.1)	
Suspect injury circumstances								
Suspect had contact with law enforcement in past 12 mo (n = 5415)	611 (11.3)	334 (14.9)	178 (8.1)	11 (9.7)	14 (11.9)	16 (21.1)	58 (8.5)	< .01
Attack believed to be direct result of suspect's mental illness (n = 5415)	442 (8.2)	289 (12.9)	91 (4.2)	15 (13.3)	4 (3.4)	8 (10.5)	35 (5.1)	< .01
Suspected substance use (other than alcohol) by suspect (n = 5415)	408 (7.5)	254 (11.4)	81 (3.7)	5 (4.4)	12 (10.2)	13 (17.1)	43 (6.3)	< .01
Suspect attempted or died by suicide after (n = 5424)	325 (6.0)	214 (9.5)	45 (2.1)	19 (16.8)	8 (6.8)	6 (7.9)	33 (4.8)	< .01
Suspect released from institutional setting within past month (n = 4364)	259 (5.9)	119 (6.6)	94 (5.3)	3 (3.3)	4 (4.4)	7 (11.1)	32 (5.6)	.2
Suspected alcohol use by suspect (n = 5415)	229 (4.2)	130 (5.8)	50 (2.3)	3 (2.7)	15 (12.7)	7 (9.2)	24 (3.5)	< .01

Note. ANHPI = Asian, Native Hawaiian, or other Pacific Islander; AIAN = American Indian or Alaska Native. We assessed racial/ethnic differences using the Bonferroni-corrected χ^2 test.
[a]Each death may have multiple suspects. However, to implement examination of suspect characteristics, we included only the primary suspect unless a different suspect was an intimate partner. If an intimate partner was listed as a suspect, we included that suspect to ensure proper intimate partner violence–related incident classification.

argument or conflict than the original study (41.5% vs 29.7%), likely because of a post-2013 change in coding guidance that allowed using this variable in conjunction with the IPV and jealousy variables.[11,17] By contrast, for non–IPV-related homicides, the original study found a higher proportion precipitated by an argument or conflict (37.8% vs 25.8%) or by a crime (41.6% vs 25.5%) than did our investigation. Further research is needed to understand drivers of these differences.

National data revealed nuanced demographic patterns across racial/ethnic groups. Homicide was the third leading cause of death for girls and women aged 15 to 24 years and the fifth leading cause of death for women aged 25 to 34 years in 2022.[4] We found that younger women accounted for higher proportions of homicides for all racial/ethnic groups except non-Hispanic White and non-Hispanic ANHPI women, which skewed middle aged and older. Similarly, 2018 to 2019 National Center for Health Statistics data showed that the homicide rate was 3.6 per 100 000 live births among pregnant and postpartum females, a 16% higher homicide rate than among nonpregnant and nonpostpartum females of reproductive age.[3] In our analysis, the proportion of women killed while pregnant or postpartum was particularly high for non-Hispanic women of 2 or more races and non-Hispanic ANHPI women (at 31.0% and 26.8% of reproductive age victims, respectively).

Homicides also had varied contexts for different racial/ethnic groups of women. Some patterns were consistent across all racial/ethnic groups: most women were killed by a firearm, and most women were fatally injured in a residence (usually their own). The suspects across groups were overwhelmingly male, underscoring the disproportionate burden of violence women experience versus perpetrate. When circumstances were known, we found that IPV accounted for almost half (47.3%) of homicides of women overall and for most homicides of non-Hispanic White, non-Hispanic ANHPI, and Hispanic women. Among IPV-related homicides, most fatal injuries across all racial/ethnic groups were inflicted by current intimate partners and an argument or conflict was the most common precipitating circumstance. Among non–IPV-related homicides, the characteristics were more varied. Some non–IPV-related commonalities across racial/ethnic groups were that the most common age group of suspects was 25 to 34 years and that argument or conflict and criminal activity were frequent precipitating circumstances.

Despite some similarities, IPV-related homicides were not uniform across racial/ethnic groups. Specific characteristics tended to be prevalent for women in different groups, such as posthomicide suicide behavior by the suspect (non-Hispanic White, non-Hispanic ANHPI), an argument or conflict (non-Hispanic Black), a history of abuse by the suspect and suspected alcohol or substance use by the suspect (non-Hispanic AIAN), prehomicide law enforcement contact with the suspect (non-Hispanic women of ≥ 2 races), and jealousy (Hispanic). These findings can be used to better understand potential sources of relationship conflict for women at risk for IPV.

Non–IPV-related homicides of women also had different circumstances across racial/ethnic groups, such as higher prevalence of family relationship problems (non-Hispanic White), drive-by shootings (non-Hispanic Black), precipitation by another crime (non-Hispanic ANHPI), precipitation by a physical fight (non-Hispanic AIAN), and relation to gangs (Hispanic). Suspects' characteristics and behaviors also differed by groups: non-Hispanic ANHPI women had the highest proportion of homicides in which the victim was a parent of the suspect, in which the attack was believed to be owing to the suspect's mental illness, and in which the suspect attempted or died by suicide. Non-Hispanic AIAN women had the most non–IPV-related homicides involving suspected alcohol use by the suspect and the most homicides perpetrated by another family member or acquaintance. Non-Hispanic women of 2 or more races were killed by suspects who had most frequently had previous encounters with law enforcement, used nonalcohol substances, or been recently released from an institutional setting. Hispanic women had the highest proportion of homicides perpetrated by strangers. These findings can be used to better understand general homicide risk factors for women.

Our findings suggest that IPV and community violence are the primary drivers of homicides of women. IPV can be chronic and continue for years, affecting lifelong health and well-being. Negative mental, physical, and economic IPV consequences are well documented,[18,19] and some findings indicate worse outcomes for marginalized groups of women, particularly related to gynecological and reproductive health.[20] Community violence occurs "in public places, such as streets or parks, between people who may or may not know each other."[21] Community violence strains the educational, justice, and medical systems and limits business growth.[22,23] Additionally, community violence has been associated with chronic disease and negative physical health outcomes,[24] and neighborhood safety concerns may cause some people to opt out of healthy behaviors.[25] We also found that non–IPV-related domestic or familial violence was common. Women were killed by family members in more than a third of non–IPV-related homicides.

Preventing violence against women could have widespread public benefits given the connection between homicides of women and other violent deaths. About a quarter of the homicide incidents that we examined were multiple fatality incidents. By contrast, when examining all 2022 NVDRS data, only 7.4% of homicide incidents included multiple fatalities.[8] We found that posthomicide suspect suicide and suicide attempts were common, particularly in IPV-related incidents. Other research has also found connections of homicides of women and IPV to mass homicides and shootings.[10,26,27] One study found that 24% of mass shooters between 1966 and 2023 targeted a specific woman in their attack.[26] Thus, effective homicide prevention for women might also prevent other violent deaths, such as mass homicides.

Limitations

This investigation was subject to limitations. The NVSS and NVDRS data covered slightly different populations, as the Web-based Injury Statistics Query and Reporting System NVSS data did not include Puerto Rico. NVDRS did not include the same jurisdictions for all data years, and some jurisdictions had data from only certain counties, rather than statewide data. These data are also limited to the information contained in their source documents. For instance, misclassifications of race and ethnicity have been documented and would be reflected in NVSS and NVDRS.[28,29]

Similarly, pregnancy status is known to be frequently misclassified or unknown on death certificates,[30] and this would be reflected in the NVDRS data and data missingness. For example, a study of 2016 data from 4 state health departments found that 38.2% of death certificates of women confirmed as pregnant via data linkage with other sources did not have a positive pregnancy checkbox marked, and most (63%) of those false negatives were owing to the checkbox being marked as "unknown" and 4% being blank.[30] Additionally, circumstance and suspect information were not available for every record. Therefore, both IPV-related and non–IPV-related homicides may be undercounted.

Public Health Implications

Our analysis uncovered characteristics that were common in homicides of women across racial/ethnic groups, most notably the high proportion of deaths involving firearms, as well as male suspects, IPV, and home environments as the injury location. Each of these characteristics could be explored for potential interventions across groups of women. Importantly, violence is multifaceted and affects different populations in different ways. Therefore, preventive interventions tailored to specific populations and communities may be beneficial.

The CDC developed the *Intimate Partner Violence Prevention Resource for Action*, outlining prevention programs at the community and societal levels based on the best available evidence.[31] The CDC's *Community Violence Prevention Resource for Action* may also be particularly relevant for the prevention of non–IPV-related homicides.[21] Primary prevention strategies such as those described in the *Resources for Action* are key to reducing violence. The examination of homicides of women by race/ethnicity provides data that can be used to efficiently and cost-effectively support these prevention efforts by focusing on the issues most relevant to homicide within communities. AJPH

ABOUT THE AUTHORS

Kaitlin Forsberg, Katherine A. Fowler, Shane P. D. Jack, and Janet M. Blair are with the Division of Violence Prevention, National Center for Injury Prevention and Control, US Centers for Disease Control and Prevention (CDC), Atlanta, GA. Bridget H. Lyons was with the Division of Violence Prevention, National Center for Injury Prevention and Control, CDC, Atlanta, GA, at the time of this study.

CORRESPONDENCE

Correspondence should be sent to Kaitlin Forsberg, Division of Violence Prevention, National Center for Injury Prevention and Control, US Centers for Disease Control and Prevention, 4770 Buford Highway, Mailstop S106-10, Atlanta, GA 30341 (e-mail: kforsberg@cdc.gov). Reprints can be ordered at https://www.ajph.org by clicking the "Reprints" link.

PUBLICATION INFORMATION

Full Citation: Forsberg K, Fowler KA, Lyons BH, Jack SPD, Blair JM. Racial/Ethnic differences in homicides of adult women and the role of intimate partner violence: United States, 2018–2022. *Am J Public Health*. 2026;116(6):829–840.

Acceptance Date: February 2, 2026.

DOI: https://doi.org/10.2105/AJPH.2026.308461

ORCID iDs:

Kaitlin Forsberg https://orcid.org/0000-0002-5779-2446

Katherine A. Fowler https://orcid.org/0000-0002-7734-1407

Bridget H. Lyons https://orcid.org/0000-0003-1152-9439

Shane P. D. Jack https://orcid.org/0000-0002-3029-0163

CONTRIBUTORS

K. Forsberg conducted the analysis and provided initial data interpretations. K. A. Fowler and B. H. Lyons conducted analysis verification. S. P. D. Jack and J. M. Blair supported data quality checking. J. M. Blair conceptualized the study. All authors contributed to the study design, drafting, editing, and final approval.

ACKNOWLEDGMENTS

Contributors to this report included participating Violent Death Reporting System programs based in US states, territories, and jurisdictions; participating jurisdiction agencies, including jurisdiction health departments, vital registrars' offices, coroners' and medical examiners' offices, crime laboratories; and local and jurisdiction law enforcement agencies.

Note. The findings and conclusions in this report are those of the authors and do not necessarily represent the official position of the Centers for Disease Control and Prevention/Agency for Toxic Substances and Disease Registry.

CONFLICTS OF INTEREST

The authors have no conflicts of interest to disclose.

HUMAN PARTICIPANT PROTECTION

This activity was reviewed by the Centers for Disease Control and Prevention (CDC) and deemed not to be human participants research. It was conducted consistently with applicable federal law and CDC policy.

REFERENCES

1. World Health Organization. Violence against women prevalence estimates, 2018: global, regional and national prevalence estimates for intimate partner violence against women and global and regional prevalence estimates for non-partner sexual violence against women. 2021. Available at: https://iris.who.int/server/api/core/bitstreams/f89348bf-8587-455a-8887-39db200f08fc/content. Accessed March 4, 2026.
2. Centers for Disease Control and Prevention. About underlying cause of death, 2018–2024, single race. Available at: https://wonder.cdc.gov/ucd-icd10-expanded.html. Accessed September 4, 2025.
3. Wallace M, Gillispie-Bell V, Cruz K, Davis K, Vilda D. Homicide during pregnancy and the postpartum period in the United States, 2018–2019. *Obstet Gynecol.* 2021;138(5):762–769. [Erratum in: Obstet Gynecol. 2022 Feb 1;139(2):347. https://doi.org/10.1097/AOG.0000000000004671]. https://doi.org/10.1097/AOG.0000000000004567
4. Centers for Disease Control and Prevention. WISQARS: Web-based injury statistics query and reporting system. Available at: https://wisqars.cdc.gov. Accessed March 1, 2024.
5. Waller BY, Joseph VA, Keyes KM. Racial inequities in homicide rates and homicide methods among Black and White women aged 25–44 years in the USA, 1999–2020: a cross-sectional time series study. *Lancet.* 2024;403(10430):935–945. https://doi.org/10.1016/S0140-6736(23)02279-1
6. Adhia A, Kernic MA, Hemenway D, Vavilala MS, Rivara FP. Intimate partner homicide of adolescents. *JAMA Pediatr.* 2019;173(6):571–577. https://doi.org/10.1001/jamapediatrics.2019.0621
7. Bush AM. A multi-state examination of the victims of fatal adolescent intimate partner violence, 2011–2015. *J Inj Violence Res.* 2020;12(1):73–83. https://doi.org/10.5249/jivr.v12i1.1197
8. Centers for Disease Control and Prevention. Surveillance for violent deaths—National Violent

Death Reporting System, 50 states, the District of Columbia, and Puerto Rico, 2022. *MMWR Surveill Summ.* 2025;74(5):1–42. https://doi.org/10.15585/mmwr.ss7405a1

9. Smith SG, Fowler KA, Niolon PH. Intimate partner homicide and corollary victims in 16 states: National Violent Death Reporting System, 2003–2009. *Am J Public Health.* 2014;104(3):461–466. https://doi.org/10.2105/AJPH.2013.301582
10. Fowler KA, Leavitt RA, Betz CJ, Yuan K, Dahlberg LL. Examining differences between mass, multiple, and single-victim homicides to inform prevention: findings from the National Violent Death Reporting System. *Inj Epidemiol.* 2021;8(1):49. https://doi.org/10.1186/s40621-021-00345-7
11. Petrosky E, Blair JM, Betz CJ, et al. Racial and ethnic differences in homicides of adult women and the role of intimate partner violence—United States, 2003–2014. *MMWR Morb Mortal Wkly Rep.* 2017;66(28):741–746. https://doi.org/10.15585/mmwr.mm6628a1
12. Heron M. Comparability of race-specific mortality data based on 1977 versus 1997 reporting standards. *Natl Vital Stat Rep.* 2021;70(3):1–31.
13. Centers for Disease Control and Prevention. Publications and information products from the National Center for Health Statistics. March 14, 2018. Available at: https://www.cdc.gov/nchs/products/index.htm. Accessed June 7, 2024.
14. Klein RJ, Schoenborn CA. Age adjustment using the 2000 projected US population. *Healthy People 2000 Stat Notes.* 2001;(20):1–9.
15. Centers for Disease Control and Prevention. About coding schemes. December 13, 2022. Available at: https://csams.cdc.gov/nioccs/HelpCodingSchemes.aspx. Accessed March 4, 2026.
16. Centers for Disease Control and Prevention. NCHS urban–rural classification scheme for counties. September 17, 2024. Available at: https://www.cdc.gov/nchs/data-analysis-tools/urban-rural.html. Accessed June 7, 2024.
17. Centers for Disease Control and Prevention. *National Violent Death Reporting System: Web Coding Manual. Version 6.1.* Available at: https://www.cdc.gov/nvdrs/media/pdfs/2025/03/nvdrs-coding-manual-version-6.1_508.pdf. Accessed March 9, 2026.
18. Peterson C, Kearns MC, McIntosh WL, et al. Lifetime economic burden of intimate partner violence among US adults. *Am J Prev Med.* 2018;55(4):433–444. https://doi.org/10.1016/j.amepre.2018.04.049
19. Leemis RW, Friar N, Khatiwada S, et al. The National Intimate Partner and Sexual Violence Survey: 2016/2017 report on intimate partner violence. October 2022. Available at: https://www.cdc.gov/nisvs/documentation/NISVSReportonIPV_2022.pdf. Accessed March 4, 2026.
20. Stockman JK, Hayashi H, Campbell JC. Intimate partner violence and its health impact on ethnic minority women [corrected]. *J Womens Health (Larchmt).* 2015;24(1):62–79. [Erratum in: *J Womens Health (Larchmt).* 2015;24(3):256. https://doi.org/10.1089/jwh.2014.4879.cxn]. https://doi.org/10.1089/jwh.2014.4879
21. Centers for Disease Control and Prevention. *Community Violence Prevention. Resource for Action: A Compilation of the Best Available Evidence for Youth and Young Adults.* Atlanta, GA: Centers for Disease Control and Prevention. 2024. Available at: https://www.cdc.gov/violence-prevention/media/pdf/resources-for-action/CV-Prevention-Resource-for-Action_508.pdf. Accessed March 4, 2026.
22. Peterson C, Aslam MV, Rice KL, Gupta N, Kearns MC. Systematic review of per person violence costs. *Am J Prev Med.* 2024;66(2):342–350. https://doi.org/10.1016/j.amepre.2023.08.009
23. McCollister KE, French MT, Fang H. The cost of crime to society: new crime-specific estimates for policy and program evaluation. *Drug Alcohol Depend.* 2010;108(1–2):98–109. https://doi.org/10.1016/j.drugalcdep.2009.12.002
24. Wright AW, Austin M, Booth C, Kliewer W. Systematic review: exposure to community violence and physical health outcomes in youth. *J Pediatr Psychol.* 2017;42(4):364–378. https://doi.org/10.1093/jpepsy/jsw088
25. Meyer OL, Castro-Schilo L, Aguilar-Gaxiola S. Determinants of mental health and self-rated health: a model of socioeconomic status, neighborhood safety, and physical activity. *Am J Public Health.* 2014;104(9):1734–1741. https://doi.org/10.2105/AJPH.2014.302003
26. Lankford A, Silva JR. Public mass shooters who target specific women: an empirical analysis of target-offender relationships, timing, and key characteristics. *Violence Against Women.* 2025. https://doi.org/10.1177/10778012251329370
27. Silva JR, Capellan JA, Schmuhl MA, Mills CE. Gender-based mass shootings: an examination of attacks motivated by grievances against women. *Violence Against Women.* 2021;27(12–13):2163–2186. https://doi.org/10.1177/1077801220981154
28. Appel NS, Edgar HJH, Berry SD, Hunley K. Error and bias in race and ethnicity descriptions in medical examiner records in New Mexico: consequences for understanding mortality among Hispanic/Latinos. *Forensic Sci Int Synerg.* 2023;7:100338. https://doi.org/10.1016/j.fsisyn.2023.100338
29. Arias E, Heron M; National Center for Health Statistics; Hakes J; US Census Bureau. The validity of race and Hispanic-origin reporting on death certificates in the United States: an update. *Vital Health Stat 2.* 2016;(172):1–21.
30. Catalano A, Davis NL, Petersen EE, et al. Pregnant? Validity of the pregnancy checkbox on death certificates in four states, and characteristics associated with pregnancy checkbox errors. *Am J Obstet Gynecol.* 2020;222(3):269.e1–269.e8. https://doi.org/10.1016/j.ajog.2019.10.005
31. Niolon PH, Kearns M, Dills J, et al. Intimate partner violence prevention. Resource for action: a compilation of the best available evidence. 2017. Available at: https://www.cdc.gov/violence prevention/pdf/IPV-Prevention-Resource_508.pdf. Accessed March 4, 2026.

Food Security by Racial and Ethnic Identity Among Lower-Income Adults

Justin T. Denney, PhD

Objectives. To expand the understanding of food security among a racially and ethnically diverse sample of US adults living below 200% of the federal poverty line (FPL).

Methods. I performed a cross-sectional analysis of the National Health Interview Survey (2019–2023) that included 37 748 respondents. I estimated unadjusted proportions and adjusted probabilities of food security for non-Hispanic White, Black, American Indian/Alaska Native (AIAN), Asian, and Hispanic adults living in severe (< 50% FPL), moderate (50% to < 100% FPL), and near poverty (100% to < 200% FPL).

Results. The study reveals important nuances in food security by race and ethnicity. Non-Hispanic Asian adults in severe poverty experienced higher food security than their counterparts in less dire economic situations, non-Hispanic Whites and Hispanics were more similar than previously reported, and non-Hispanic AIAN adults reported extremely low probabilities of food security.

Conclusions. Thoroughly documenting and expanding on these patterns of food security for lower-income adults could lead to better understanding of policy mechanisms that could alleviate food insecurity and reduce health disparities by racial and ethnic identity in the United States. (*Am J Public Health*. 2026;116(6):841–850. https://doi.org/10.2105/AJPH.2026.308508)

AJPH June 2026, Vol. 116, No. 6

Food insecurity is defined as a household-level social and economic condition that includes a lack of access to adequate food for a healthy, active lifestyle.[1] In the United States, it is a major public health issue and has been widely recognized as such for several decades.[2–5] Its association with poor health is multipronged, affecting consumption patterns that lead to the development of chronic conditions such as heart disease and diabetes.[3] Food-insecure individuals also often delay medical care and alter prescribed medication use to purchase food.[6,7] Doing so leads to cascading poorer health outcomes and emergency care, often accompanied by expensive and sometimes lengthy hospital stays.[6,7]

Despite efforts to improve food security, many American households suffer from inadequate access to food. Low income is a leading contributor, and research has rightfully concentrated on this risk factor and how to alleviate food insecurity in the face of economic challenges. In 2023, over 13% of all US households were food insecure, and nearly 3 times that proportion (> 38%) with incomes below the federal poverty line (FPL; according to the US Department of Health and Human Services) were food insecure.[1] However, this also means that the majority of poor households are food secure. Undoubtedly, many existing social service programs, including the Supplemental Nutrition Assistance Program (SNAP) and the Women, Infants, and Children (WIC) program effectively address food insecurity among poorer families.[2] Participation in these programs is not as high as it could be for households that qualify. For example, scholars describe nonparticipation in SNAP for eligible families resulting from things like stigma associated with receiving benefits and the transaction costs of recertifying eligibility if a family temporarily stops receiving benefits but later wants to reenroll.[8] Consequently, scholars have called for better understanding of the characteristics and possible coping strategies employed to achieve food security in challenging social and economic conditions.[8]

Food security has many well-identified sociodemographic and socioeconomic patterns. Older adults in the United States report more food security than younger adults,[9,10] food security is higher among men than women,[10] and it is higher for married adults compared with never married and divorced or separated adults.[11] Food security is also often lower in households that include children compared with households without children because families struggle to accommodate nutritional needs for children and adults.[9]

Income has a well-documented positive relationship with food security. In 2023, significantly more households with an income at or above 185% of the FPL reported food security (92.5%) compared with the national average (86.5%).[12] At the same time, households below the poverty line are considerably less likely to be food secure. In 2023, only 62% of these households reported food security.[12] Beyond income, food security is also positively associated with higher levels of educational attainment and current employment.[9]

Ample research has shown the benefits of SNAP for low-income households in terms of alleviating food insecurity.[8] Nevertheless, food security rates tend to be lower in households receiving SNAP, as SNAP reflects the neediest families and those at highest risk of food insecurity. When selection into SNAP is accounted for, the benefits of SNAP in helping families avoid food insecurity become evident.[13]

There is limited research on regional and rural–urban differences in food insecurity. In 2023, food insecurity for rural households (15.4%) slightly exceeded that for all US households (13.5%).[12] Recent work has provided insights into rural–urban differences in food security when broken down by region of the United States. A recent study used unique data on services provided in rural and urban areas across the United States and showed that high charitable food-related services, such as food banks, made a measurable difference in addressing food insecurity in remote rural areas.[14]

Finally, a large body of research has documented differences in food security by racial and ethnic identity. Food security is less prevalent in households headed by non-Hispanic Black and Hispanic adults compared with non-Hispanic White households.[9,10,15,16] (Hereafter, all racial/ethnic groups are non-Hispanic unless otherwise indicated.) A recent study focused on nativity found lower rates of food security for immigrant and native-born Blacks and Hispanics compared with Whites.[15] More detailed differences in food security by race and ethnicity are largely unavailable because of data restrictions. For example, the annual food security report produced by the US Department of Agriculture (USDA) does show that Asian adults tend to have the highest rates of food security,[12] but the reports do not include estimates for American Indian/Alaska Native (AIAN) individuals, nor does the recent Census Household Pulse Survey.[17] Although nationally representative estimates are limited, smaller-scale studies do indicate lower food security for AIAN individuals.[17,18]

The current study had 2 primary objectives. First, it investigated food security among lower-income adults (≤ 200% of the FPL) to examine differences by more and less economically challenged lower-income adults. Below 200% of the FPL is used by many social service programs to define "low-income" eligibility.[19] Second, the study aimed to illuminate detailed differences in food security by racial and ethnic identity among this lower-income sample. The majority of existing studies, although not examining detailed levels of poverty, generally (though not always the case for all groups) depict lower food security for racial and ethnic minorities, compared with Whites.[9,10,15,16] If income is a uniform driving factor behind food security, then food security should be highest for the full sample and for all racial and ethnic groups in the highest income group of the sample. (In the current study, the near-poor group [100% to ≤ 200% of FPL] is the highest income group.) If that is not the case, it suggests that either social services are not uniformly reaching groups or being evenly utilized across groups[8,20,21] or there are unique strategies some groups may employ to enhance food security in challenging economic circumstances.[22–25]

METHODS

The IPUMS National Health Interview Survey (NHIS) provided the data used here for adults aged 25 years and older who were below 200% of the FPL. Publicly available data can be downloaded from https://nhis.ipums.org/nhis. The sampling strategy for the NHIS changed in 2019, so all analyses here used 2019–2023 data, the latest years available at the time of analysis.[26] Comparisons before and after 2018 using the NHIS are not recommended.[26]

Food security was measured in this study using the USDA's adult food security survey module (https://www.ers.usda.gov/topics/food-nutrition-assistance/food-security-in-the-us/survey-tools), which includes 10 items. The items are yes/no queries on topics such as (1) worried that food would run out before there was money to buy more and (2) couldn't afford to eat balanced meals.[26] Affirmative responses to 0 items indicate high food security, 1 or 2 items marginal

AJPH June 2026, Vol. 116, No. 6

food security, 3 to 5 items low food security, and 6 or more items very low food security. Over 86% of the NHIS lower-income respondents identifying as food secure (≤ 2 affirmative responses) were high food secure (0 affirmative responses), and fewer than 6% of the respondents were very low food secure. Because the current study aimed to investigate food security by poverty and racial/ethnic identity, examining more detailed food security statuses was restricted by sample considerations. Following established convention, the analyses proceeded by classifying adults responding affirmatively to 2 or fewer of the 10 items as food secure, whereas 3 or more items resulted in food insecure classification.[1]

Poverty was measured as the ratio of family income to the US Census Bureau's poverty thresholds specific to survey year completion. This allowed comparisons for adults in severe poverty (< 50% of FPL), moderate poverty (50% to < 100% of FPL), and near poverty (100% to < 200% of FPL). For race/ethnicity, I classified respondents into 6 groups: White, Black, AIAN, Asian, other, and Hispanic.

A number of sociodemographic and socioeconomic control variables relevant for food security status were included. Age was measured continuously, and an age-squared term was included in regression analyses to accommodate the nonlinear association of age with food security, as indicated by model goodness-of-fit statistics.[27] Gender was a binary indicator (female and male); food stamp receipt was a binary indicator of whether the respondent received benefits from SNAP; marital status included married, divorced or separated, widowed, cohabiting, and never married; household composition was included as a binary indicator of whether there were children younger than 18 years in the household; nativity included whether the respondent was born in the United States; educational attainment included high school or less, some college, and bachelor's degree or more; employment status was a binary indicator of currently employed or not; region of the United States captured the residence of the respondent as the Northeast, Midwest and Central, South, and West; and a binary indicator captured whether the adult lives in a rural county.

To better understand food security for lower-income adults, I retained the sample below 200% of the FPL in the NHIS for analysis. Most items in the NHIS had very low percentages of missing data. A total of 592 cases (1.6% of the lower-income sample) missing data on food security, age, gender, household composition, education, or a combination of these covariates were dropped (missingness on each of these individual measures was ≤ 1%). Roughly 4.5% to 5.5% of the individual measures for food stamp receipt, marital status, nativity, and employment were missing data. To maximize the sample and reduce bias, I included a missing category for these covariates. All analyses are weighted and adjusted for the complex sampling design of the NHIS using Stata software.[28]

To address the objectives of the analysis, unadjusted weighted percentage differences in food security are provided for all covariates for the full sample and within the categories of poverty. Next, a logistic regression model reports odds ratios for food security, adjusting for all covariates. I determined goodness-of-fit with the recommended *F*-adjusted test statistic and associated *P* value for survey adjusted logistic regression.[27] Finally, I estimated predicted marginal probabilities from a fully adjusted logistic regression plus an interaction for race/ethnicity and poverty level to assess the ways in which poverty and race/ethnicity interact to affect food security.[29,30] Pairwise *t* tests of differences between predicted marginal probabilities assessed fully adjusted differences between groups.[29,30]

RESULTS

Table 1 provides information on the sample sizes and percentage of food security for the full sample and for the poverty subsamples. It also provides the percentage of food security for each sample within the categories of all covariates. Over 80% of the 37 156 low-income adults included in this study reported food security. Food security varied considerably across poverty subsamples. For example, over 84% of the 23 899 near-poverty adults reported food security and only 73.8% of the 3295 severe-poverty adults did so. For descriptive information on all covariates for the full sample and within each subsample of the poverty categories, see Table A (available as a supplement to the online version of this article at http://www.ajph.org).

By race and ethnicity, Whites (82.5%) and Hispanics (81.3%) had statistically similar percentages of food security in this lower-income sample; Asians had a statistically significantly higher percentage (87.3%) of food security than Whites; and Blacks (74.9%), AIANs (70.2%), and others (71.0%) had statistically lower proportions of food security than Whites. These patterns for the full sample were generally consistent across the categories of poverty, with a few exceptions. Statistically significantly fewer Hispanics in severe poverty (70.8%) were food secure than Whites in severe poverty (76.4%). A significantly lower percentage of AIANs in severe poverty reported food security (62.1%), and a significantly higher percentage of Asian adults in severe poverty reported food security (90.1%).

Table 1 shows other differences in food security by the covariates included in this study that were generally consistent across categories of poverty. Food-secure adults were on average older than food-insecure adults. Male respondents were more often food secure than female respondents for the full sample. The significant difference by gender, however, was only present in the near-poor category when broken down by poverty subsamples. Married adults were more often food secure than other marital statuses, except for widowed respondents. The only statistically significant difference in food security between households with and without children can be seen in the severe-poverty category, where fewer households with children (71.7%) reported food security than households without children (75.7%).

The highest educated lower-income adults in the sample were more often food secure (86.4%) than both the lowest educated (80.1%) and those with some college education (79.7%). Employed adults were also more often food secure (81.9%) than those not working (78.2%). There were very few differences geographically and no differences between adults in rural counties versus nonrural counties.

Adjusted Odds of Food Security

Table 2 provides fully adjusted odds ratios for food security. An assessment of the independent variables in Table 2 (minus the quadratic for age) produced variance inflation factors that did not exceed 2.5, providing no evidence of multicollinearity.[31] The adjusted estimates are similar to patterns from Table 1. Regarding poverty and race/ethnicity, adults in the most severe and the moderate categories of poverty, compared with adults in the near-poverty category, had significantly lower adjusted odds of food security. By racial and ethnic identity, Black, AIAN, and other adults had significantly lower adjusted odds of food security, compared with Whites. Asians had significantly higher adjusted odds than Whites, and Hispanics were statistically indistinguishable from Whites in their adjusted odds of food security.

Intersection of Racial/Ethnic Identity by Level of Poverty

Figure 1 presents predicted probabilities generated from the fully adjusted logistic regression models from Table 2 plus an interaction between poverty level and race. The letters in the figure represent significance ($P \le .05$) from pairwise statistical tests of differences in the probabilities.[29,30]

First, Figure 1a shows that Whites in severe poverty were (1) statistically significantly more likely food secure than AIANs and Hispanics in severe poverty and (2) statistically indistinguishable from Blacks. They were also less likely than Asians in this level of poverty to be food secure. In fact, Asian adults in severe poverty had a probability of food security of 0.89, statistically significantly greater than that of any other group. The fully adjusted probability of food security for AIAN adults in severe poverty was 0.67 and statistically significantly lower than for Whites, Blacks, and Asians.

There were overall fewer significant differences by race in the moderate poverty category. The probability of food security for Whites was significantly greater than for Blacks and others but indistinguishable from that for all other groups, including Asians.

More differences existed in the near-poverty category by race and ethnicity (Figure 1a). Fully adjusted probabilities for food security for Whites were greater than for Blacks, AIANs, and others. Near-poor Blacks and AIANs were also statistically less likely than near-poor Asians and Hispanics to be food secure. Near-poor Whites were statistically similar to near-poor Asians and Hispanics in their probability of food security.

If income was a uniform driving factor behind food security, Figure 1b should show a pattern of increasing probability of food security moving from severe to near poverty for each of the racial and ethnic groups. There is some evidence of that notion, but also some discrepancies. As shown in Figure 1b, among the near poor, only Whites and Hispanics were statistically more likely to be food secure than adults in more dire economic circumstances. There were, however, no statistical differences between severe- and moderate-poverty White and Hispanic adults. Likely partly because of sample restraints, there were no differences between poverty categories for AIANs. Finally, counterintuitively, Asians in severe poverty had statistically significantly higher food security likelihoods than their counterparts in moderate poverty. The probability of food security for severe-poor Asian adults (0.89) also exceeded the probability for their near-poor counterparts (0.86), but that difference did not reach statistical significance.

TABLE 1— Unadjusted Percentages of Food Security and Tests of Differences Between Categories of Covariates for the Full Sample and by Subsamples of Poverty Status: United States, 2019–2023

	All Adults	Severe Poverty	Moderate Poverty	Near Poverty
Full and subsample, No.	37 156	3 295	9 962	23 899
Food security, %				
Secure	80.7***	73.8***	74.4***	84.2***
Insecure	19.3	26.2	25.6	15.8
Poverty, %				
Severe (< 50% FPL)	73.8***	...	...	...
Poor (50% to < 100% FPL)	74.4***	...	...	...
Near (100% to < 200% FPL) (Ref)	84.2	...	...	...
Race/ethnicity, %				
Non-Hispanic White (Ref)	82.5	76.4	75.0	85.6
Non-Hispanic Black	74.9***	71.2*	70.3**	78.0***
Non-Hispanic AIAN	70.2**	62.1***	69.6	73.6*
Non-Hispanic Asian	87.3***	90.1***	82.4**	88.8**
Non-Hispanic other	71.0***	65.1	64.6*	75.1***
Hispanic	81.3	70.8*	75.8	85.4
Food secure age, y, mean	52.3***	48.0**	51.6***	53.1***
Food insecure age, y, mean	48.9	46.1	49.9	48.9
Gender, %				
Male	82.0***	75.8	75.5	85.1**
Female	79.8	72.6	73.6	83.4
SNAP receipt, %				
Yes	70.0***	65.4***	67.8***	73.2***
No (Ref)	85.1	80.3	78.7	86.9
Missing	98.3***	97.6***	97.5***	98.9***
Marital status, %				
Married (Ref)	83.6	77.0	76.1	86.4
Divorced/separated	74.0***	61.3***	66.9***	79.8***
Widowed	85.1*	73.3	79.8*	88.2*
Cohabitating	75.3***	71.5	71.4*	77.3***
Never married	76.9***	73.5	71.9*	80.2***
Missing	98.6***	99.8***	97.6***	98.8***
Children younger than 18 y in household, %				
Yes	80.6	71.7*	75.2	84.4
No	80.8	75.7	73.7	84.0
Born in the United States, %				
Yes (Ref)	79.1	73.1	71.6	82.7
No	81.7***	69.9	76.1***	85.9***
Missing	98.6***	98.6***	98.5***	98.6***
Educational attainment, %				
High school or less (Ref)	80.1	71.5	74.0	84.1
Some college	79.7	74.6	72.3	82.8
Bachelor's degree or more	86.4***	85.1***	83.5***	87.3***

Continued

AJPH June 2026, Vol. 116, No. 6

TABLE 1— Continued

	All Adults	Severe Poverty	Moderate Poverty	Near Poverty
Employment status, %				
Employed (Ref)	81.9	76.8	76.5	83.9
Not employed	78.2***	69.5***	70.9***	83.2
Missing	99.7***	99.4***	99.7***	99.8***
Region, %				
Northeast (Ref)	81.9	72.7	73.8	86.2
Midwest	80.0	74.5	73.9	82.9**
South	79.8*	73.0	73.1	83.5**
West	82.4	75.6	77.7*	84.9
Rural county, %				
Yes	81.0	74.0	73.8	85.2
No	80.6	73.7	74.5	83.9

Note. AIAN = American Indian/Alaska Native; FPL = federal poverty line (according to the US Department of Health and Human Services); SNAP = Supplemental Nutrition Assistance Program. The sample comprised adults aged ≥ 25 years living below 200% of the FPL. Tests of significant differences were determined by a *z* test for proportions (*t* test for mean differences). Percentages are representative of the proportion of individuals in each covariate category who were food secure.
Source. National Health Interview Survey, 2019–2023.[26]
*$P \le .05$; **$P \le .01$; ***$P \le .001$.

DISCUSSION

Several insights into racial and ethnic differences in food security arise by looking at a lower-income sample of Americans. It is often reported that racial minority groups, particularly Blacks and Hispanics, are less often food secure than Whites.[9,10,15,16] The current study finds that probabilities of food security for lower-income adults in the United States are more nuanced. As important illustrations, the probability of food security for Whites is greater than among Hispanics only for those adults in severe poverty (≤ 50% of FPL). For moderate and near-poor adults, food security probabilities are similar to those for Whites and Hispanics. Furthermore, Asians in severe poverty have some of the highest levels of food security of the entire sample, higher than for Asians with more economic resources. In addition, the adjusted

TABLE 2— Fully Adjusted Logistic Regression of Food Security: United States, 2019–2023

	OR (95% CI)
Poverty	
Near (Ref)	1
Severe (< 50% FPL)	0.73 (0.65, 0.82)
Poor (50% to < 100% FPL)	0.71 (0.66, 0.77)
Race/ethnicity	
Non-Hispanic White (Ref)	1
Non-Hispanic Black	0.74 (0.67, 0.82)
Non-Hispanic AIAN	0.57 (0.37, 0.87)
Non-Hispanic Asian	1.22 (0.99, 1.50)
Non-Hispanic other	0.59 (0.48, 0.74)
Hispanic	0.95 (0.85, 1.07)
Age	0.89 (0.88, 0.91)
Age squared	1.01 (1.01, 1.01)
Gender	
Female (Ref)	1
Male	1.11 (1.04, 1.19)
SNAP receipt	
No (Ref)	1
Yes	0.54 (0.50, 0.59)
Missing	2.52 (1.50, 4.22)

Continued

TABLE 2— Continued

	OR (95% CI)
Marital status	
Married (Ref)	1
Divorced/separated	0.71 (0.65, 0.79)
Widowed	0.81 (0.70, 0.93)
Cohabitating	0.76 (0.67, 0.87)
Never married	0.95 (0.85, 1.06)
Missing	1.10 (0.56, 2.16)
Children younger than 18 y in household	
No (Ref)	1
Yes	1.41 (1.29, 1.55)
Born in the United States	
No (Ref)	1
Yes	1.01 (0.90, 1.13)
Missing	1.11 (0.48, 2.57)
Educational attainment	
High school or less (Ref)	1
Some college	1.00 (0.92, 1.08)
Bachelor's degree or more	1.38 (1.23, 1.56)
Employment status	
Not employed (Ref)	1
Employed	1.39 (1.28, 1.51)
Missing	32.18 (7.49, 138.17)
Region	
Northeast (Ref)	1
Midwest	0.88 (0.77, 1.00)
South	0.91 (0.81, 1.02)
West	1.00 (0.88, 1.14)
Rural county	
No (Ref)	1
Yes	1.13 (1.01, 1.27)
F-adjusted test statistic	0.71
P	.7

Note. AIAN = American Indian/Alaska Native; CI = confidence interval; FPL = federal poverty line (according to the US Department of Health and Human Services); OR = odds ratio; SNAP = Supplemental Nutritional Assistance Program. The sample comprised adults aged ≥ 25 years living below 200% of the FPL. All models controlled for year of survey. The total sample was 37 156.
Source. National Health Interview Survey, 2019–2023.[26]

probability of food security for Whites and Blacks is similar for adults living in severe poverty, whereas for those in moderate and near poverty, Whites are more likely to be food secure than Blacks.

Very few studies at the national level have included AIANs. In the current study, AIANs, particularly those in the severe- and near-poor categories, experienced significantly lower food security than many other groups. For example, AIANs living in severe poverty were statistically less likely (adjusted probability = .67) than Whites, Blacks, and Asians to be food secure. Previous research has indicated that the health consequences of food insecurity are greater for racial and ethnic minorities.[32,33] This seems particularly salient for AIANs given the disadvantages in food security documented here. Food security is a major public health issue for all adults, and it may go a long way toward explaining persistent health disparities for AIAN adults.[17,18]

Limitations

There are noteworthy limitations of the current work. First, there is a need to further delineate Hispanic groups. Previous health disparities research has shown the important heterogeneity among Hispanic/Latine groups,[34] and food security research should follow suit when samples allow. This is also an important consideration among Asian subgroups.[35] Second, the current study is largely descriptive but provides evidence that racial and ethnic groups may be employing diverse and unique strategies to avoid food insecurity.[22–25] More in-depth studies are needed to illuminate what these strategies are, and why, when, and for whom they might be effective in reducing food insecurity.

Public Health Implications

The patterns of difference in food security by race/ethnicity and level of poverty reported here suggest at least 2 possibilities. On the one hand, services that can help assist with food security may be more unevenly experienced or delivered among low-income adults. Research shows important differences in the uptake of food assistance services among needy families[8] and suggests, for example, targeted efforts to increase participation among

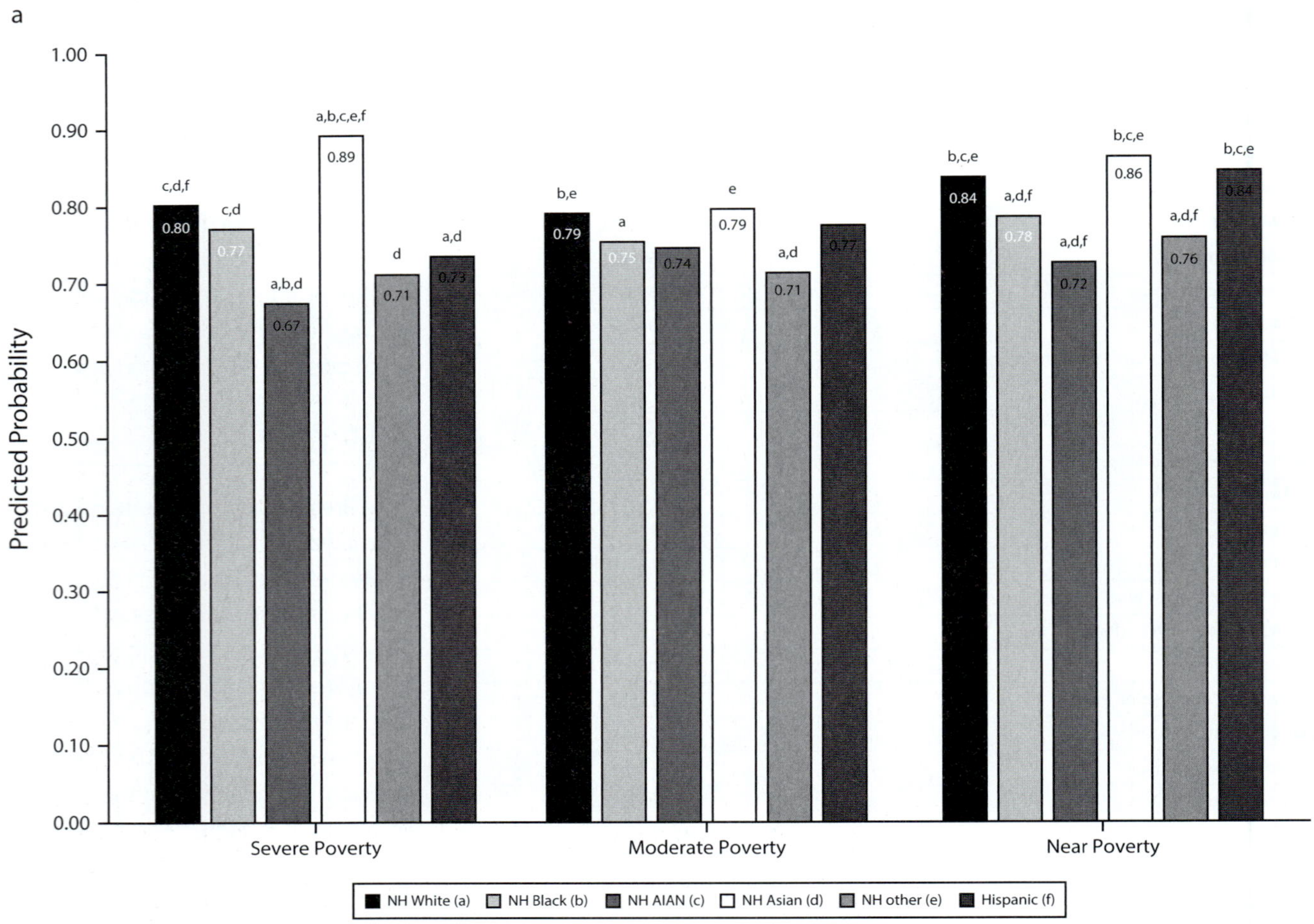

FIGURE 1— **Predicted Probability of Food Security by (a) Race/Ethnicity Within Poverty Categories and (b) Poverty Status Within Race/Ethnicity Categories: United States, 2019–2023**

Note. The figure shows fully adjusted predicted marginal probabilities of food security derived from the logistic regression in Table 2 plus an interaction between poverty and race/ethnicity. Goodness-of-fit for the interaction model was assessed using the *F*-adjusted test statistic[27] ($F = 0.89$) with a *P* value of .53, indicating adequate fit. An adjusted Wald *F* test provides evidence that the interaction improves model fit over the model without interaction provided in Table 2 (adjusted $F = 13.14$, $P \le .001$). Letters in the figure indicate statistical significance at the $P \le .05$ level for postestimation pairwise comparisons of the predicted marginal probabilities (i.e., contrasts) within poverty level and between racial and ethnic identities (a) and within racial and ethnic identity and between poverty levels (b). Significance for the contrasts is determined by a *t* test of difference using the delta method for standard errors.[29,30]

the most vulnerable groups.[20] SNAP includes work requirements, and research has shown that these contribute to uneven participation by race/ethnicity.[21] Work requirements for SNAP have recently expanded (see https://www.fns.usda.gov/snap/work-requirements), creating the potential for even greater disparities in participation by race/ethnicity.

On the other hand, the ways in which families interact with their communities to maintain food security in challenging financial situations may include more and less effective strategies. Evidence for this notion comes from recent research showing strong positive associations between the cohesiveness of communities and food security,[22,23,25] above and beyond individual- and family-level factors important for food security. A study based in California revealed considerable differences across racial and ethnic groups in the benefits of a cohesive community.[23] Perceived community cohesion in this study showed no impact on food security for Asians and progressively larger positive impacts for Whites, Blacks, and Hispanics.[23]

Although presented as 2 distinct possibilities, it is likely that benefits from food assistance access and participation and socially cohesive communities simultaneously enhance food security. However, they may do

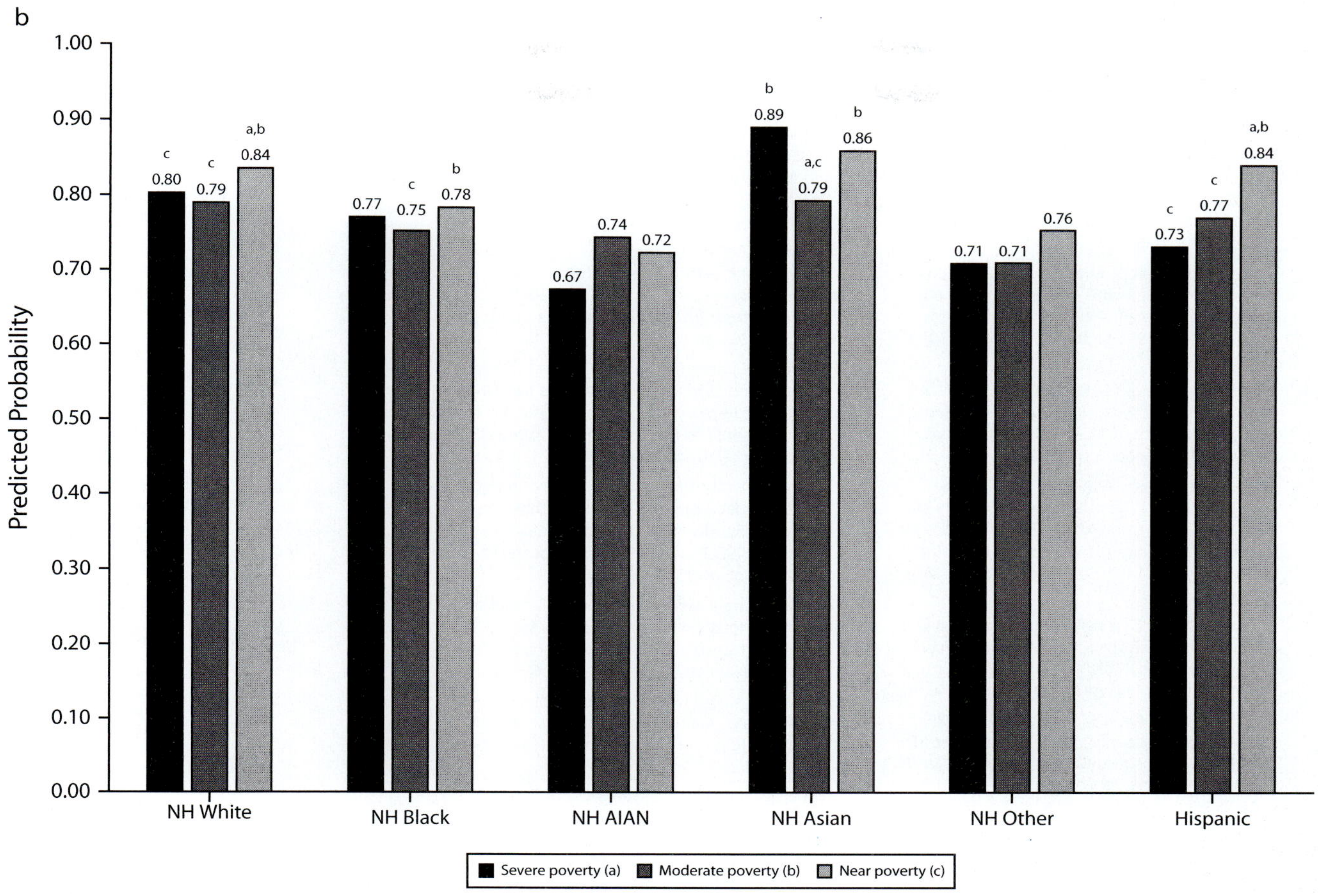

FIGURE 1— Continued

so synergistically for some groups whereas one or the other may have negligible impacts for other groups. Expanding the understanding of racial and ethnic patterns of food security for lower-income adults could lead to policy mechanisms that might alleviate food insecurity and reduce health disparities by racial and ethnic identity in the United States. AJPH

ABOUT THE AUTHOR

Justin T. Denney is with the Department of Sociology, Washington State University, Pullman.

CORRESPONDENCE

Correspondence should be sent to Justin Denney, 100 Dairy Rd, Department of Sociology, Washington State University, Pullman, WA 99164-4020 (e-mail: justin.denney@wsu.edu). Reprints can be ordered at https://www.ajph.org by clicking the "Reprints" link.

PUBLICATION INFORMATION

Full Citation: Denney JT. Food security by racial and ethnic identity among lower-income adults. *Am J Public Health*. 2026;116(6):841–850.

Acceptance Date: February 17, 2026.

DOI: https://doi.org/10.2105/AJPH.2026.308508

ORCID iD:
Justin T. Denney https://orcid.org/0000-0003-0246-4004

ACKNOWLEDGMENTS

I thank the William Julius Wilson Distinguished Professorship and the Department of Sociology at Washington State University for supporting this research.

CONFLICTS OF INTEREST

The author has no conflicts of interest to declare.

HUMAN PARTICIPANT PROTECTION

This study was deemed exempt by the Washington State University institutional review board. All data used are public-use secondary data available for download at https://nhis.ipums.org/nhis.

REFERENCES

1. US Dept of Agriculture, Economic Research Service. Food security and nutrition assistance. 2025. Available at: https://www.ers.usda.gov/data-products/ag-and-food-statistics-charting-the-essentials/food-security-and-nutrition-assistance. Accessed December 1, 2025.
2. Gundersen C, Ziliak JP. Food insecurity and health outcomes. *Health Aff (Millwood)*. 2015; 34(11):1830–1839. https://doi.org/10.1377/hlthaff.2015.0645
3. Murthy VH. Food insecurity: a public health issue. *Public Health Rep*. 2016;131(5):655–657. https://doi.org/10.1177/0033354916664154
4. Bruening M, MacLehose R, Loth K, Story M, Neumark-Sztainer D. Feeding a family in a recession: food insecurity among Minnesota parents. *Am J Public Health*. 2012;102(3): 520–526. https://doi.org/10.2105/AJPH.2011.300390
5. Stuff JE, Casey PH, Szeto KL, et al. Household food insecurity is associated with adult health status. *J Nutr*. 2004;134(9):2330–2335. https://doi.org/10.1093/jn/134.9.2330

6. Herman D, Afulani P, Coleman-Jensen A, Harrison GG. Food insecurity and cost-related medication underuse among nonelderly adults in a nationally representative sample. *Am J Public Health.* 2015;105(10):e48–e59. https://doi.org/10.2105/AJPH.2015.302712
7. Berkowitz SA, Seligman HK, Choudhry NK. Treat or eat: food insecurity, cost-related medication underuse, and unmet needs. *Am J Med.* 2014;127(4):303–310.e303. https://doi.org/10.1016/j.amjmed.2014.01.002
8. Gundersen C, Ziliak JP. Food insecurity research in the United States: where we have been and where we need to go. *Applied Eco Perspectives Pol.* 2018;40(1):119–135. https://doi.org/10.1093/aepp/ppx058
9. Gundersen C, Kreider B, Pepper J. The economics of food insecurity in the United States. *Applied Eco Perspectives Pol.* 2011;33(3):281–303. https://doi.org/10.1093/aepp/ppr022
10. Walker RJ, Garacci E, Dawson AZ, Williams JS, Ozieh M, Egede LE. Trends in food insecurity in the United States from 2011–2017: disparities by age, sex, race/ethnicity, and income. *Popul Health Manag.* 2021;24(4):496–501. https://doi.org/10.1089/pop.2020.0123
11. Hanson KL, Sobal J, Frongillo EA. Gender and marital status clarify associations between food insecurity and body weight. *J Nutr.* 2007;137(6):1460–1465. https://doi.org/10.1093/jn/137.6.1460
12. Rabbitt MP, Reed-Jones M, Hales LJ, Burke MP. Household food security in the United States in 2023. US Dept of Agriculture, Economic Research Service. 2024. https://doi.org/10.32747/2024.8583175.ers
13. Gundersen C, Kreider B, Pepper J, Tarasuk V. Food assistance programs and food insecurity: implications for Canada in light of the mixing problem. *Empir Econ.* 2017;52(3):1065–1087. https://doi.org/10.1007/s00181-016-1191-4
14. Gundersen C, Dewey A, Hake M, Engelhard E, Crumbaugh AS. Food insecurity across the rural–urban divide: are counties in need being reached by charitable food assistance? *Ann Am Acad Pol Soc Sci.* 2017;672(1):217–237. https://doi.org/10.1177/0002716217710172
15. Myers AM, Painter MA. Food insecurity in the United States of America: an examination of race/ethnicity and nativity. *Food Sec.* 2017;9(6):1419–1432. https://doi.org/10.1007/s12571-017-0733-8
16. Hales LJ, Coleman-Jensen A. *Household Food Security Across Race and Ethnicity in the United States, 2016–21.* Kansas City, MO: US Dept of Agriculture, Economic Research Service; 2024. Report No. EIB-269.
17. Nikolaus CJ, Johnson S, Benally T, et al. Food insecurity among American Indian and Alaska Native people: a scoping review to inform future research and policy needs. *Adv Nutr.* 2022;13(5):1566–1583. https://doi.org/10.1093/advances/nmac008
18. Blue Bird Jernigan V, Wetherill MS, Hearod J, et al. Food insecurity and chronic diseases among American Indians in rural Oklahoma: the THRIVE study. *Am J Public Health.* 2017;107(3):441–446. https://doi.org/10.2105/AJPH.2016.303605
19. US Dept of Health and Human Services. Poverty Guidelines. Office of the Assistant Secretary for Planning and Evaluation. Available at: https://aspe.hhs.gov/..topics/poverty-economic-mobility/poverty-guidelines. Accessed August 7, 2025.
20. Miller DP, Nepomnyaschy L, Ibarra GL, Garasky S. Family structure and child food insecurity. *Am J Public Health.* 2014;104(7):e70–e76. https://doi.org/10.2105/AJPH.2014.302000
21. Brantley E, Pillai D, Ku L. Association of work requirements with Supplemental Nutrition Assistance Program participation by race/ethnicity and disability status, 2013–2017. *JAMA Netw Open.* 2020;3(6):e205824. https://doi.org/10.1001/jamanetworkopen.2020.5824
22. Denney JT, Brewer M, Kimbro RT. Food insecurity in households with young children: a test of contextual congruence. *Soc Sci Med.* 2020;263:113275. https://doi.org/10.1016/j.socscimed.2020.113275
23. Denney JT, Kimbro RT, Heck K, Cubbin C. Social cohesion and food insecurity: insights from the Geographic Research on Wellbeing (GROW) Study. *Matern Child Health J.* 2017;21(2):343–350. https://doi.org/10.1007/s10995-016-2119-5
24. Denney JT, Kimbro RT, Sharp G. Neighborhoods and food insecurity in households with young children: a disadvantage paradox? *Social Problems.* 2018;65(3):342–359. https://doi.org/10.1093/socpro/spw054
25. King C. Informal assistance to urban families and the risk of household food insecurity. *Soc Sci Med.* 2017;189:105–113. https://doi.org/10.1016/j.socscimed.2017.07.030
26. Blewett LA, Rivera Drew JA, King ML, et al. *IPUMS Health Surveys: National Health Interview Survey, Version 7.4* [data set]. Minneapolis, MN: IPUMS; 2024.
27. Archer KJ, Lemeshow S. Goodness-of-fit test for a logistic regression model fitted using survey sample data. *Stata J.* 2006;6(1):97–105. https://doi.org/10.1177/1536867X0600600106
28. *Stata Statistical Software: Release 18* [computer program]. College Station, TX: Stata Corporation; 2024.
29. Long JS, Mustillo SA. Using predictions and marginal effects to compare groups in regression models for binary outcomes. *Sociol Methods Res.* 2021;50(3):1284–1320. https://doi.org/10.1177/0049124118799374
30. Mize TD. Best practices for estimating, interpreting, and presenting nonlinear interaction effects. *Sociol Sci.* 2019;6:81–117. https://doi.org/10.15195/v6.a4
31. Vittinghoff E, Shiboski SC, Glidden DV, McCulloch CE. *Regression Methods in Biostatistics: Linear, Logistic, Survival, and Repeated Measures Models.* New York, NY: Springer; 2005.
32. Walker RE, Keane CR, Burke JG. Disparities and access to healthy food in the United States: a review of food deserts literature. *Health Place.* 2010;16(5):876–884. https://doi.org/10.1016/j.healthplace.2010.04.013
33. Odoms-Young A, Brown AG, Agurs-Collins T, Glanz K. Food insecurity, neighborhood food environment, and health disparities: state of the science, research gaps and opportunities. *Am J Clin Nutr.* 2024;119(3):850–861. https://doi.org/10.1016/j.ajcnut.2023.12.019
34. Lebron CN, Borrell LN. Pa'Lante, Pa'tras ni Para Coger Impulso: the future of Hispanic or Latino Health and Research. *Am J Public Health.* 2024;114(S6):S420–S421. https://doi.org/10.2105/AJPH.2024.307769
35. Yom S, Lor M. Advancing health disparities research: the need to include Asian American subgroup populations. *J Racial Ethn Health Disparities.* 2022;9(6):2248–2282. https://doi.org/10.1007/s40615-021-01164-8

Trends in Meningococcal B Vaccine Uptake Among 16- and 17-Year-Old Adolescents in the United States: An Analysis of the National Immunization Survey–Teen, 2018–2023

Neeta P. Regmi, MPH, MBBS, Tiankai Xie, MS, Angela K. Ulrich, PhD, MPH, and Nicole E. Basta, PhD, MPhil

Objectives. To examine trends in meningococcal B (MenB) vaccination coverage among US adolescents aged 16 and 17 years.

Methods. We conducted cross-sectional and longitudinal analyses of 2018 to 2023 National Immunization Survey–Teen data to calculate the annual percentage of eligible adolescents who received the MenB vaccine and to assess changes over time.

Results. Only 19.8% of the 41 505 eligible adolescents initiated MenB vaccination between 2018 and 2023. A total of 24.5% (95% confidence interval [CI] = 22.5, 26.6) of adolescents received 1 or more MenB vaccinations in 2023, as compared with 13.2% (95% CI = 11.7, 14.6) in 2018. Among initiators, most received only 1 dose.

Conclusions. MenB vaccination coverage among 16- and 17-year-old adolescents increased modestly between 2018 and 2023. As of 2023, approximately 3 out of 4 adolescents in this age group had not received the MenB vaccine.

Public Health Implications. As of 2023, less than one quarter of 16- and 17-year-old adolescents had initiated MenB vaccination. Given that MenB has accounted for most meningococcal disease among adolescents and young adults since 2013, efforts to improve uptake are warranted. (*Am J Public Health*. 2026;116(6):851–854. https://doi.org/10.2105/AJPH.2026.308459)

AJPH June 2026, Vol. 116, No. 6

Meningococcal disease is a rare but important public health concern in the United States because of its outbreak potential and high case-fatality rate of approximately 15%.[1] Adolescents are at increased risk for infection, and group B accounted for the majority of all meningococcal cases among adolescents and young adults between 2013 and 2022.[2] In 2022, fewer than one third of 17-year-old adolescents received at least 1 dose of the meningococcal B (MenB) vaccine.[3]

The MenB vaccine was first approved for use in the United States in 2014.[4] In 2015, the Advisory Committee on Immunization Practices (ACIP) recommended MenB vaccination for individuals 16 to 23 years old on the basis of shared clinical decision-making.[5] Beginning in 2017, the recommended MenB dosing schedules for adolescents not at increased risk were 2 doses of MenB vaccine, either MenB-4C (Bexsero) administered at least 1 month apart or 2 doses of MenB-FHbp (Trumenba) administered 6 months apart.[6] In 2023, the pentavalent meningococcal vaccine (MenACWY-TT/MenB-FHbp) was recommended for use when both MenACWY and MenB were indicated at the same visit, potentially simplifying coadministration and improving uptake.[7] In 2024, ACIP recommended that both MenB-4C and MenB-FHbp be administered in

2 doses 6 months apart (ideally between the ages of 16 and 18 years) on the basis of shared clinical decision-making.[8] We assessed annual MenB vaccine uptake among adolescents 16 to 17 years of age in the United States from 2018 to 2023 to establish baseline coverage estimates in the years preceding the 2024 recommendation changes.

METHODS

The National Immunization Survey–Teen (NIS–Teen) is an annual, cross-sectional survey designed to monitor vaccination coverage among US adolescents 13 to 17 years of age.[9] Data are collected from both parents and health care providers, but information on MenB vaccination status is collected only from providers. Participants whose health care providers have reported their vaccination status for each vaccine are classified by NIS–Teen as having "adequate provider data." NIS–Teen study methods and complete documentation are available online.[10]

Eligibility

We assessed annual MenB vaccination coverage among 2018 to 2023 NIS–Teen participants 16 to 17 years of age who were living in the United States and had adequate provider data, including MenB vaccination status (Figure A, available as a supplement to the online version of this article at http://www.ajph.org).

Statistical Analysis

MenB vaccination status was based on health care provider reports, with participants who received at least 1 dose of MenB vaccine classified as having initiated vaccination; all reported doses were included regardless of vaccine brand and were included even if the provider did not report the brand ("unspecified MenB type"). We applied NIS–Teen survey weights to all of our analyses because they were designed to generate nationally representative estimates by accounting for potential sociodemographic differences between those with and without adequate provider data and by addressing potential nonresponse bias. Initially, we assessed the demographic characteristics of participants eligible for our analysis. We then calculated the annual weighted percentages of adolescents 16 to 17 years of age who had received (1) 1 or more doses of MenB vaccine, (2) only 1 MenB vaccine dose (i.e., those who had initiated but had not completed the recommended 2-dose series by the time of the survey), and (3) 2 or more doses (i.e., those who had completed at least the recommended 2 doses by the time of the survey).

To statistically assess temporal trends in vaccination coverage, we fitted a survey-weighted logistic regression model using survey year as a continuous predictor and receipt of at least 1 MenB vaccine dose as the binary outcome. All of the variables included in our analysis are described in Table B (available as a supplement to the online version of this article at http://www.ajph.org). Statistical analyses were conducted with R version 4.4.1 (R Foundation for Statistical Computing, Vienna, Austria).

RESULTS

Overall, 41 505 adolescents met the eligibility criteria and were included in our analyses. Demographic characteristics were similar across years, with slightly more 16-year-old than 17-year-old participants and slightly more male than female participants. The majority of participants identified as non-Hispanic White, more than one third resided in the southern region, and most had private insurance (Table C, available as a supplement to the online version of this article at http://www.ajph.org).

Across all years, 19.8% of participants received at least 1 dose of any MenB vaccination. Initiation of MenB vaccination increased between 2018 and 2023. Annual vaccination rates for 1 or more doses of MenB vaccine were 13.2% (95% confidence interval [CI] = 11.7%, 14.6%) in 2018, 16.2% (95% CI = 14.5%, 18.0%) in 2019, 20.7% (95% CI = 18.9%, 22.6%) in 2020, 23.0% (95% CI = 20.9%, 25.1%) in 2021, 22.4% (95% CI = 20.6%, 24.3%) in 2022, and 24.5% (95% CI = 22.5%, 26.6%) in 2023 (Figure 1 and Table 1).

Correspondingly, the percentage of adolescents who were unvaccinated at the time of the survey declined from 86.8% (95% CI = 85.4%, 88.3%) in 2018 to 75.5% (95% CI = 73.4%, 77.5%) in 2023. There was a significant increase in the percentage of adolescents initiating MenB vaccination from 2018 to 2023 (annual odds ratio [OR] = 1.15; 95% CI = 1.12, 1.18). The percentage who completed the 2-dose MenB series was lower than the percentage who had received only 1 dose by the time of the survey. Among those who had initiated vaccination, 39.7% (95% CI = 33.6%, 45.9%) completed the 2-dose series in 2018, as compared with 36.9% (95% CI = 32.3%, 41.5%) in 2023 (Table D, available as a supplement to the online version of this article at http://www.ajph.org).

DISCUSSION

Our multiyear assessment provides an updated overview of MenB vaccine uptake among adolescents 16 to 17 years

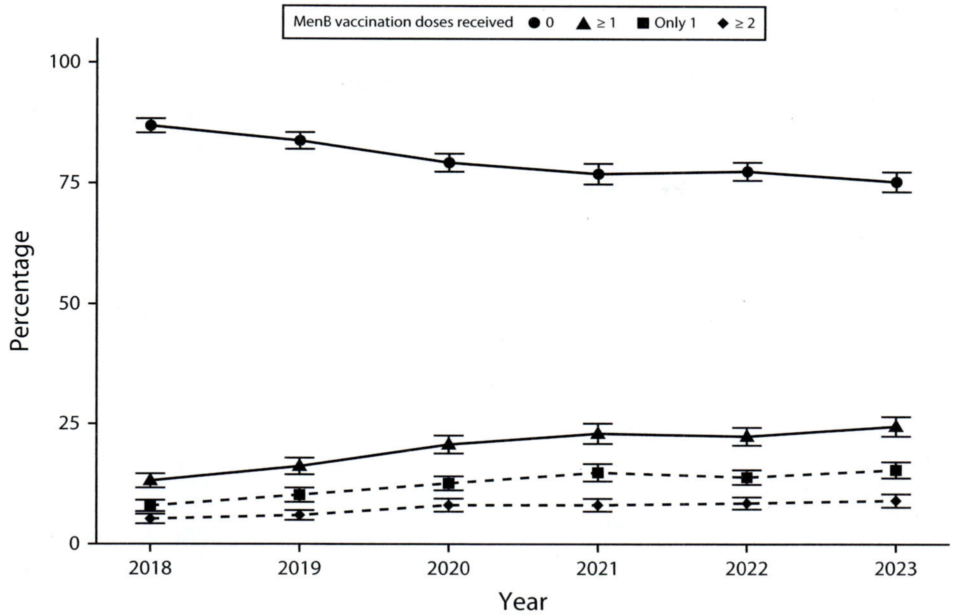

FIGURE 1— **Distribution of Percentage of 16- and 17-Year-Old National Immunization Survey–Teen Participants by Number of Doses of Meningococcal B Vaccine Received: United States, 2018–2023**

of age. In our analysis, we found that the percentage of adolescents initiating the MenB vaccine series increased from 13.2% to 24.5% between 2018 and 2023. However, in 2023, most participants who initiated the series received 1 dose; only 36.9% reported completing the recommended 2-dose series. The majority of adolescents did not receive a MenB vaccine according to annual estimates from 2018 through 2023.

However, given that NIS–Teen vaccination status reflects vaccinations only at the time of the survey and that participants were 16 to 17 years old, participants could have initiated or completed the MenB vaccine series after the survey while they still remained eligible for vaccination, making our estimates of vaccination series completion likely conservative. We focused on adolescents starting at the age of 16 years on the basis of the ACIP recommendation that the ideal age for MenB vaccination is 16 to 18 years.

Previous NIS–Teen analyses from 2023 indicated that 32.4% of adolescents had initiated MenB vaccination (as compared with 24.5% in our study). Our estimates differ because earlier analyses included 17-year-old adolescents only and excluded vaccinations in which the MenB vaccine type was unknown. We took a more comprehensive approach, including adolescents beginning at 16 years of age (consistent with ACIP recommendations), including provider-reported MenB doses in which the vaccine type was unspecified,[11] and conducting longitudinal analyses.

TABLE 1— **Distribution of Percentage of 16- and 17-Year-Old National Immunization Survey–Teen Participants by Number of Doses of Meningococcal B Vaccine Received: United States, 2018–2023**

No. of Doses	2018, % (95% CI)	2019, % (95% CI)	2020, % (95% CI)	2021, % (95% CI)	2022, % (95% CI)	2023, % (95% CI)
0	86.8 (85.4, 88.3)	83.8 (82.0, 85.5)	79.3 (77.4, 81.1)	77.0 (74.9, 79.1)	77.6 (75.7, 79.4)	75.5 (73.4, 77.5)
≥ 1	13.2 (11.7, 14.6)	16.2 (14.5, 18.0)	20.7 (18.9, 22.6)	23.0 (20.9, 25.1)	22.4 (20.6, 24.3)	24.5 (22.5, 26.6)
1[a]	7.9 (6.8, 9.1)	10.2 (8.7, 11.7)	12.6 (11.2, 14.1)	14.9 (13.1, 16.7)	13.9 (12.4, 15.5)	15.5 (13.8, 17.2)
≥ 2[a]	5.2 (4.2, 6.2)	6.0 (5.0, 7.0)	8.1 (6.7, 9.4)	8.1 (6.8, 9.4)	8.5 (7.3, 9.8)	9.0 (7.7, 10.4)

Note. CI = confidence interval. The sample size was 41 505.
[a]Percentages were calculated among all eligible participants. The percentage who received only 1 dose and the percentage who received ≥ 2 doses equal the percentage who received ≥ 1 doses.

Of note, our 2018 to 2023 uptake estimates reflect pre-2024 vaccination recommendations. Future research examining MenB vaccination disparities, equity, and barriers (e.g., related to visit timing and access); investigating comparisons with MenACWY coverage; and evaluating interventions designed to improve adolescent vaccination is warranted, especially as recommendations change.

In summary, MenB vaccination coverage among 16- to 17-year-old adolescents increased modestly between 2018 and 2023. As of 2023, approximately 3 out of 4 adolescents in this age group had not received the MenB vaccine. Vaccination remains the most effective strategy for reducing the risk of MenB disease.

PUBLIC HEALTH IMPLICATIONS

As of 2023, fewer than 1 in 4 adolescents 16 to 17 years of age had initiated MenB vaccination. Given that MenB has accounted for most meningococcal cases among adolescents and young adults since 2013, preventing MenB disease among adolescents remains an important public health priority. AJPH

ABOUT THE AUTHORS

Neeta P. Regmi is with the Division of Environmental Health Sciences, School of Public Health, University of Minnesota, Minneapolis. Tiankai Xie is with the Department of Bioinformatics and Computational Biology, College of Science and Engineering, University of Minnesota, Minneapolis. Angela K. Ulrich is with the Center for Infectious Disease Research and Policy, University of Minnesota, Minneapolis. Nicole E. Basta is with the Division of Epidemiology, Biostatistics, and Occupational Health, School of Population and Global Health, Faculty of Medicine and Health Sciences, McGill University, Montreal, Quebec, Canada.

CORRESPONDENCE

Correspondence should be sent to Neeta P. Regmi, MPH, MBBS, Division of Environmental Health Sciences, School of Public Health, University of Minnesota, 1260 Mayo Building, MMC 807, 420 Delaware St SE, Minneapolis, MN 55455 (e-mail: pokhr020@umn.edu). Reprints can be ordered at https://www.ajph.org by clicking the "Reprints" link.

PUBLICATION INFORMATION

Full Citation: Regmi NP, Xie T, Ulrich AK, Basta NE. Trends in meningococcal B vaccine uptake among 16- and 17-year-old adolescents in the United States: an analysis of the National Immunization Survey–Teen, 2018–2023. *Am J Public Health*. 2026;116(6):851–854.

Acceptance Date: February 1, 2026

DOI: https://doi.org/10.2105/AJPH.2026.308459

ORCID iDs:

Neeta P. Regmi https://orcid.org/0009-0000-4842-8522

Tiankai Xie https://orcid.org/0000-0001-5729-9734

CONTRIBUTORS

N. P. Regmi contributed to the conception and design of the study, conducted analyses, interpreted the results, and wrote the article. T. Xie conducted analyses and revised the article critically for important intellectual content. A. K. Ulrich contributed to the conception and design of the study and revised the article critically for important intellectual content. N. E. Basta originated the study, contributed to the design of the study and interpretation of results, and revised the article critically for important intellectual content. All of the authors reviewed the final version.

ACKNOWLEDGMENTS

Nicole E. Basta is supported by a Canadian Institutes of Health Research Canada Research Chair in Infectious Disease Prevention.

CONFLICTS OF INTEREST

The authors have no conflicts of interest to declare.

HUMAN PARTICIPANT PROTECTION

This study involved a secondary analysis of deidentified, publicly available data and was exempt from institutional review board oversight.

REFERENCES

1. US Centers for Disease Control and Prevention. Meningococcal disease. Available at: https://www.cdc.gov/surv-manual/php/table-of-contents/chapter-8-meningococcal-disease.html. Accessed January 28, 2025.
2. Mbaeyi SA, Bozio CH, Duffy J, et al. Meningococcal vaccination: recommendations of the Advisory Committee on Immunization Practices, United States, 2020. *MMWR Recomm Rep.* 2020;69(9):1–41. https://doi.org/10.15585/mmwr.rr6909a1
3. Pingali C, Yankey D, Elam-Evans LD, et al. Vaccination coverage among adolescents aged 13–17 years—National Immunization Survey–Teen, United States, 2022. *MMWR Morb Mortal Wkly Rep.* 2023;72(34):912–919. https://doi.org/10.15585/mmwr.mm7234a3
4. US Centers for Disease Control and Prevention. Use of serogroup B meningococcal vaccines in persons aged ≥10 years at increased risk for serogroup B meningococcal disease: recommendations of the Advisory Committee on Immunization Practices, 2015. *MMWR Morb Mortal Wkly Rep.* 2015;64(22):610–613.
5. MacNeil JR, Rubin L, Folaranmi T, Ortega-Sanchez IR, Patel M, Martin SW. Use of serogroup B meningococcal vaccines in adolescents and young adults: recommendations of the Advisory Committee on Immunization Practices, 2015. *MMWR Morb Mortal Wkly Rep.* 2015;64(41):1171–1176. https://doi.org/10.15585/mmwr.mm6441a3
6. Patton ME, Stephens D, Moore K, MacNeil JR. Updated recommendations for use of MenB-FHbp serogroup B meningococcal vaccine—Advisory Committee on Immunization Practices, 2016. *MMWR Morb Mortal Wkly Rep.* 2017;66(19):509–513. https://doi.org/10.15585/mmwr.mm6619a6
7. Collins JP, Crowe SJ, Ortega-Sanchez IR, et al. Use of the Pfizer pentavalent meningococcal vaccine among persons aged ≥10 years: recommendations of the Advisory Committee on Immunization Practices—United States, 2023. *MMWR Morb Mortal Wkly Rep.* 2024;73(15):345–350. https://doi.org/10.15585/mmwr.mm7315a4
8. Schillie S, Loehr J, Chen WH, et al. New dosing interval and schedule for the Bexsero MenB-4C vaccine: updated recommendations of the Advisory Committee on Immunization Practices—United States, October 2024. *MMWR Morb Mortal Wkly Rep.* 2024;73(49):1124–1128. https://doi.org/10.15585/mmwr.mm7349a3
9. US Centers for Disease Control and Prevention. About the National Immunization Surveys. Available at: https://www.cdc.gov/nis/about/index.html. Accessed January 25, 2025.
10. US Centers for Disease Control and Prevention. NIS-Teen data and documentation for 2015 to present. Available at: https://www.cdc.gov/nis/php/datasets-teen/index.html. Accessed January 20, 2025.
11. Pingali C, Yankey D, Chen M, et al. National vaccination coverage among adolescents aged 13–17 years—National Immunization Survey–Teen, United States, 2023. *MMWR Morb Mortal Wkly Rep.* 2024;73(33):708–714. https://doi.org/10.15585/mmwr.mm7333a1

Prevalence of Multiple Chronic Conditions Among US Adults, 2024

Lindsey I. Black, MPH, Amanda E. Ng, PhD, MPH, Benjamin Zablotsky, PhD, and Brian W. Ward, PhD

Objectives. To provide current prevalence estimates for diagnosed multiple chronic conditions (MCC) among the noninstitutionalized, civilian US adult population.

Methods. We analyzed data from the 2024 National Health Interview Survey (n = 32 629) to produce estimates and population counts for adults with 0, 1, or 2 or more conditions by demographic characteristics.

Results. In 2024, 51.1% of US adults had at least 1 of 10 selected diagnosed chronic conditions, and 26.4% had MCC. Variations in the prevalence of MCC were observed by sex, race and Hispanic origin, age, health insurance coverage, and urbanization level.

Conclusions. The National Health Interview Survey can be used to provide timely estimates on population prevalence of MCC. Prevalence of MCC in 2024 was similar to that of 2010 estimates, and subgroup differences have persisted. Results may inform public health efforts and guide prevention strategies aimed at addressing multiple chronic conditions among adults in the US population. (*Am J Public Health*. 2026;116(6):855–858. https://doi.org/10.2105/AJPH.2026.308427)

AJPH June 2026, Vol. 116, No. 6

Chronic health conditions are a significant public health concern that are costly to manage, contribute to excess health care utilization, and decrease health-related quality of life.[1–4] Chronic conditions affect more than three quarters of US adults, with prevalence rising in recent years, especially among young adults.[5]

Previous reports have used data from the National Health Interview Survey (NHIS) to produce prevalence estimates for single chronic conditions and multiple chronic conditions (MCC) among US adults based on 10 selected diagnosed chronic conditions (arthritis, cancer, chronic obstructive pulmonary disease, coronary heart disease, current asthma, diabetes, hepatitis, hypertension, stroke, and weak or failing kidneys).[6–8] They have shown that the prevalence varied across sociodemographic characteristics. The prevalence of MCC was higher among women, increased with age, and was higher among non-Hispanic White and Black adults compared with Hispanic and Asian adults. Among adults aged younger than 65 years, the prevalence of MCC varied by health insurance coverage and tended to be higher among those with public health insurance, while among adults aged 65 years or older, the prevalence was highest among those with Medicare and Medicaid ("dual eligible"). Rural areas also had higher rates of chronic conditions compared with urban areas.

In this study, we used 2024 NHIS data to update these estimates and describe differences in prevalence by selected sociodemographic characteristics. In addition, we examined changes in the prevalence of MCC from the 2010 and 2024 NHIS.

METHODS

We used data from the 2024 NHIS to estimate the prevalence of MCC among selected chronic conditions for adults aged 18 years and older (n = 32 629).[9] The NHIS is an annual, cross-sectional household survey representative of the civilian, noninstitutionalized US population. NHIS is a survey of a subset of the US population and uses a multistage, stratified cluster sampling design to achieve national representativeness. One adult per household is randomly selected to respond to a detailed health interview covering a broad range of topics, including chronic conditions.

Interviews are typically initiated face to face in respondents' homes, with follow-ups conducted over the telephone. Because households are sampled and there is the potential for participants that are selected to not go on to participate (e.g., the 2024 final response rate was 47.9% among adults), sample weights are created to account for this nonresponse and allow for the production of nationally representative estimates.

Consistent with previous reports,[6–8] we selected 10 conditions from a list of 20, developed by the US Department of Health and Human Services, to foster a standardized approach of measuring the occurrence of chronic conditions.[10] In NHIS, adults reported if they had ever been told by a doctor or health care provider that they had arthritis, cancer, chronic obstructive pulmonary disease (including emphysema and chronic bronchitis), coronary heart disease, diabetes, hepatitis, hypertension, or stroke, or that they currently had asthma. Adults were categorized as having 0, 1, or 2 or more of these conditions. Additional chronic conditions are measured in NHIS on a periodic basis; however, we selected these 10 to be consistent with previous reports[6–8] and to allow for exploration of temporal changes in the prevalence of MCC between survey years. We examined selected demographics of sex, race and Hispanic origin, age group, current health insurance coverage, and urbanization level. Urbanization was based on the 2023 National Center for Health Statistics (NCHS) urban–rural classification scheme for counties.[11] We generated estimates and 95% Korn–Graubard confidence intervals (CIs) by using SUDAAN version 11.0.1 (RTI International, Research Triangle Park, NC) to account for the NHIS complex sample design. All estimates met NCHS reliability standards.[12] Crude prevalence and population estimates are presented. We used the 2-tailed *t* test ($P < .05$) to evaluate significant differences by sociodemographic subgroups and to examine changes in the prevalence of MCC between the 2010 and 2024 NHIS.

RESULTS

In 2024, 51.1% (approximately 133 million) of civilian, noninstitutionalized US adults had at least 1 of the 10 selected diagnosed chronic conditions examined. In total, 24.7% (approximately 64 million) of adults had 1 chronic condition, while 26.4% (approximately 69 million) US adults had MCC (Table 1). The prevalence of MCC was higher among women (27.1%) compared with men (25.7%). The prevalence of MCC was highest for non-Hispanic White adults (29.7%) compared with Hispanic adults (16.7%), non-Hispanic Asian adults (17.8%), and non-Hispanic other or multiple race adults (22.3%); however, the prevalence for non-Hispanic White adults was not significantly different from non-Hispanic Black adults (29.3%) or non-Hispanic American Indian/Alaska Native adults (28.7%). Prevalence of MCC increased with age, with 62.0% of adults aged 65 years and older having MCC compared with 6.4% of those aged 18 to 44 years. Among adults aged 18 to 64 years, the prevalence of MCC was highest among those with public insurance (22.5%), while among adults aged 65 years and older, the prevalence was highest among those with both Medicare and Medicaid ("dual eligible"; 72.3%). Adults living in nonmetropolitan areas had a higher prevalence of MCC (34.7%) compared with those living in any of the other urbanization levels. The prevalence of MCC among all adults did not change significantly ($P = .41$) between 2010 (26.0%) and 2024 (data not shown).

DISCUSSION

According to NHIS data on 10 selected conditions, approximately 1 in 4 US adults (26.4%) had MCC in 2024. This is not a significant change from previous estimates of diagnosed MCC among US adults for the same 10 conditions in 2010 (26.0%).[8] Differences in MCC prevalence were found across selected demographic characteristics, where MCC was more common among women, adults aged 65 years and older, and adults living in rural areas. The prevalence of MCC also varied by health insurance coverage. The subgroup differences observed in 2024 have persisted from previous years that have examined MCC among US adults.[6–8]

This study is not without limitations. First, NHIS data may be subject to recall bias, as the data are based on self-report. Second, only 10 of the 20 chronic conditions outlined by the definition of the US Department of Health and Human Services were included in the analysis.[10] Third, chronic conditions measured by the NHIS are limited to adults with diagnoses and do not include undiagnosed conditions. It is important to note that the chronic conditions autism spectrum disorder, congestive heart failure, cardiac arrhythmias, dementia, depression, HIV, hyperlipidemia, osteoporosis, schizophrenia, or substance abuse disorders were not included in the current composite definition, and trends for these unmeasured conditions could differ from those observed for the included chronic diseases. Further research examining the prevalence of MCC based on the inclusion of more conditions can be explored with NHIS data in future publications. Finally,

TABLE 1— Percentage and Number of US Adults Aged 18 Years and Older With Chronic Conditions, by Select Characteristics: United States, 2024

Characteristic	0 Chronic Conditions		1 Chronic Condition		≥2 Chronic Conditions	
	% (95% CI)	Population[a]	% (95% CI)	Population[a]	% (95% CI)	Population[a]
Total[b]	48.9 (48.1, 49.7)	126 968	24.7 (24.1, 25.3)	64 096	26.4 (25.8, 27.0)	68 590
Demographics						
Sex[c]						
Male	50.2 (49.1, 51.3)	63 411	24.1 (23.3, 25.0)	30 489	25.7 (24.8, 26.6)	32 459
Female	47.7 (46.7, 48.6)	63 506	25.2 (24.4, 26.0)	33 596	27.1 (26.3, 27.9)	36 131
Race and Hispanic origin[d]						
Non-Hispanic White	44.4 (43.5, 45.3)	70 488	25.9 (25.1, 26.6)	41 047	29.7 (29.0, 30.5)	47 196
Non-Hispanic Black	45.5 (43.0, 47.9)	13 972	25.3 (23.5, 27.1)	7 769	29.3 (27.3, 31.3)	8 990
Non-Hispanic Asian	60.7 (57.8, 63.5)	9 909	21.5 (19.2, 23.9)	3 504	17.8 (15.7, 20.1)	2 912
Non-Hispanic American Indian/Alaska Native	47.4 (39.2, 55.7)	793	23.9 (17.4, 31.4)	400	28.7 (21.3, 37.1)	481
Non-Hispanic other and multiple races	54.3 (49.4, 59.1)	3 053	23.4 (19.4, 27.8)	1 316	22.3 (18.8, 26.2)	1 256
Hispanic	61.7 (59.9, 63.6)	28 752	21.6 (20.2, 23.0)	10 061	16.7 (15.3, 18.0)	7 756
Age group,[c] y						
18–44	73.8 (72.8, 74.8)	87 480	19.8 (19.0, 20.7)	23 505	6.4 (5.8, 6.9)	7 543
45–64	38.5 (37.4, 39.6)	31 231	31.9 (30.8, 33.0)	25 885	29.6 (28.5, 30.7)	24 041
≥ 65	13.5 (12.8, 14.3)	8 070	24.5 (25.8, 27.1)	14 599	62.0 (60.8, 63.1)	36 915
Health insurance coverage[e]						
18–64 y[c]						
Private	59.8 (58.8, 60.8)	82 514	25.8 (25.0, 26.6)	35 615	14.4 (13.8, 15.0)	19 855
Public	55.3 (53.0, 57.6)	16 328	22.2 (20.4, 24.2)	6 561	22.5 (20.8, 24.2)	6 630
Uninsured	70.2 (67.8, 72.5)	16 287	21.0 (18.8, 23.3)	4 872	8.8 (7.5, 10.2)	2 034
≥ 65 y[f]						
Private	14.4 (13.2, 15.7)	2 827	25.3 (23.6, 27.1)	4 969	60.2 (58.4, 62.1)	11 809
Dual eligible	8.9 (6.6, 11.7)	408	18.9 (15.7, 22.4)	867	72.3 (68.4, 75.9)	3 324
Medicare Advantage	13.2 (12.0, 14.5)	3 103	25.3 (23.7, 26.9)	5 952	61.5 (59.6, 63.4)	14 472
Medicare only excluding Medicare Advantage	18.2 (15.6, 21.0)	1 204	27.2 (24.1, 30.5)	1 800	54.6 (50.9, 58.2)	3 609
Urbanization level[c,g]						
Large central metro	54.0 (52.7, 55.2)	44 482	24.0 (22.9, 25.0)	19 740	22.1 (21.0, 23.1)	18 179
Large fringe metro	50.3 (48.8, 51.8)	32 393	24.9 (23.8, 26.1)	16 052	24.8 (23.5, 26.2)	15 976
Medium and small metro	46.7 (45.2, 48.3)	35 633	24.7 (23.6, 25.9)	18 846	28.5 (27.3, 29.7)	21 747
Nonmetropolitan	39.5 (37.8, 41.3)	14 459	25.8 (24.6, 27.1)	9 459	34.7 (33.0, 36.3)	12 688

Note. Chronic conditions included were arthritis, cancer, chronic obstructive pulmonary disease, current asthma, diabetes, heart disease, hepatitis, hypertension, stroke, and weak or failing kidneys.

[a]Population in 1000s.

[b]Total 2024 US adult population: 260 million people. Numbers may not sum to group totals because of rounding.

[c]Difference in estimates for 2 or more chronic conditions between all subcategories was significant at $P < .05$.

[d]Difference in estimates for 2 or more chronic conditions between by race and Hispanic origin show that non-Hispanic White adults were significantly different from all other race and Hispanic origin groups with the exception of non-Hispanic Black adults ($P = .65$) and non-Hispanic American Indian/Alaska Native adults ($P = .79$), non-Hispanic Black adults were significantly different from all other race and Hispanic origin groups with the exception of non-Hispanic American Indian/Alaska Native adults ($P = .89$), non-Hispanic Asian adults were significantly different from all other race and Hispanic origin groups with the exception of Hispanic adults ($P = .35$), and non-Hispanic American Indian/Alaska Native adults were significantly different from all other race and Hispanic origin groups with the exception of non-Hispanic other or multiple race adults ($P = .14$).

[e]Health insurance coverage was based on a hierarchy of mutually exclusive categories.[9]

[f]With the exception of private versus Medicare Advantage ($P = .33$), all other differences in estimates for 2 or more chronic conditions among adults aged 65 years and older by insurance status were significantly different.

[g]Linear trend was significant ($P < .001$) with decreasing urbanization level for estimates of 2 or more chronic conditions.

NHIS data are collected from a sample of the civilian, noninstitutionalized population and, therefore, are not inclusive of institutionalized adults and adults in long-term care settings, where health status may differ. For these reasons, results are an underestimate of the true population burden of chronic conditions in the United States.

This work builds upon previous research by providing updated and timely estimates of the prevalence of MCC for 10 common conditions among US adults. Its finding that 26% of adults have diagnosed MCC supports the understanding that chronic conditions continue to be a concern for the field of public health and the health care system.[1–4] These prevalence estimates can be used to inform public health efforts and help guide primary, secondary, and tertiary prevention strategies aimed at addressing MCC among the US population. AJPH

ABOUT THE AUTHORS

Lindsey I. Black, Amanda E. Ng, and Benjamin Zablotsky are with the Division of Health Interview Statistics at the National Center for Health Statistics, Hyattsville, MD. Brian W. Ward is with the Division of Health Care Statistics at the National Center for Health Statistics.

Note. All views expressed in this article are those of the authors and do not necessarily reflect those of the Centers for Disease Control and Prevention or the National Center for Health Statistics.

CORRESPONDENCE

Correspondence should be sent to Lindsey Black, National Center for Health Statistics, Room 5223, 3311 Toledo Rd, Hyattsville, MD 20782-2064 (e-mail: lblack1@cdc.gov). Reprints can be ordered at https://www.ajph.org by clicking the "Reprints" link.

PUBLICATION INFORMATION

Full Citation: Black LI, Ng AE, Zablotsky B, Ward BW. Prevalence of multiple chronic conditions among US adults, 2024. *Am J Public Health*. 2026;116(6): 855–858.

Acceptance Date: December 14, 2025.

DOI: https://doi.org/10.2105/AJPH.2026.308427

ORCID iDs:

Lindsey I. Black https://orcid.org/0000-0001-9417-069X

Amanda E. Ng https://orcid.org/0000-0002-5212-3147

Benjamin Zablotsky https://orcid.org/0000-0002-1759-3485

Brian W. Ward https://orcid.org/0000-0001-8257-1592

CONTRIBUTORS

All authors conceptualized and designed the work. L. Black and A. Ng acquired and analyzed the data. All authors contributed to interpreting the data. All authors drafted the article, revised it critically, made substantial contributions to editing the article, and approved the version to be published.

ACKNOWLEDGMENTS

The authors would like to thank Jeannine Schiller, Jessica Jones, Anjel Vahratian, Stephen Blumberg, Alexander Strashny, and Amy Branum for their support and review of the article.

CONFLICTS OF INTEREST

The authors declare no potential conflicts of interest with respect to the research, authorship, or publication of this article.

HUMAN PARTICIPANT PROTECTION

No protocol approval was necessary because the data were publicly available and lacked personal identifiers.

REFERENCES

1. Skinner HG, Coffey R, Jones J, Heslin KC, Moy E. The effects of multiple chronic conditions on hospitalization costs and utilization for ambulatory care sensitive conditions in the United States: a nationally representative cross-sectional study. *BMC Health Serv Res*. 2016;16:77–78. https://doi.org/10.1186/s12913-016-1304-y
2. Mujica-Mota RE, Roberts M, Abel G, et al. Common patterns of morbidity and multi-morbidity and their impact on health-related quality of life: evidence from a national survey. *Qual Life Res*. 2015;24(4):909–918. https://doi.org/10.1007/s11136-014-0820-7
3. Buttorff C, Ruder T, Bauman M. Multiple chronic conditions in the United States. RAND Corporation. 2017. Available at: https://www.rand.org/content/dam/rand/pubs/tools/TL200/TL221/RAND_TL221.pdf. Accessed February 1, 2025.
4. DuGoff EH, Canudas-Romo V, Buttorff C, Leff B, Anderson GF. Multiple chronic conditions and life expectancy: a life table analysis. *Med Care*. 2014;52(8):688–694. https://doi.org/10.1097/MLR.0000000000000166
5. Watson KB, Wiltz JL, Nhim K, Kaufmann RB, Thomas CW, Greenlund KJ. Trends in multiple chronic conditions among US adults, by life stage, Behavioral Risk Factor Surveillance System, 2013–2023. *Prev Chronic Dis*. 2025;22:E15. https://doi.org/10.5888/pcd22.240539
6. Ward BW, Schiller JS. Prevalence of multiple chronic conditions among US adults: estimates from the National Health Interview Survey, 2010. *Prev Chronic Dis*. 2013;10:E65. https://doi.org/10.5888/pcd10.120203
7. Ward BW, Schiller JS, Goodman RA. Multiple chronic conditions among US adults: a 2012 update. *Prev Chronic Dis*. 2014;11:E62. https://doi.org/10.5888/pcd11.130389
8. Boersma P, Black LI, Ward BW. Prevalence of multiple chronic conditions among US adults, 2018. *Prev Chronic Dis*. 2020;17:E106. https://doi.org/10.5888/pcd17.200130
9. National Center for Health Statistics. National Health Interview Survey, 2024 survey description. 2025. Available at: https://ftp.cdc.gov/pub/Health_Statistics/NCHS/Dataset_Documentation/NHIS/2024/srvydesc-508.pdf. Accessed July 17, 2025.
10. Goodman RA, Posner SF, Huang ES, Parekh AK, Koh HK. Defining and measuring chronic conditions: imperatives for research, policy, program, and practice. *Prev Chronic Dis*. 2013;10:E66. https://doi.org/10.5888/pcd10.120239
11. National Center for Health Statistics. NCHS urban–rural classification scheme for counties. Available at: https://www.cdc.gov/nchs/data-analysis-tools/urban-rural.html. Accessed May 29, 2025.
12. Parker JD, Talih M, Malec DJ, et al. National Center for Health Statistics data presentation standards for proportions. *Vital Health Stat 2*. 2017(175):1–22.

Erratum In: "Science in Service: Reflections on the MacArthur 'Genius' Fellowship"

In: Dasgupta N. Science in service: reflections on the MacArthur "Genius" Fellowship. *Am J Public Health*. 2026;116(2):157–158.

When originally published, the author's first name was spelled incorrectly.

https://doi.org/10.2105/AJPH.2025.308375e

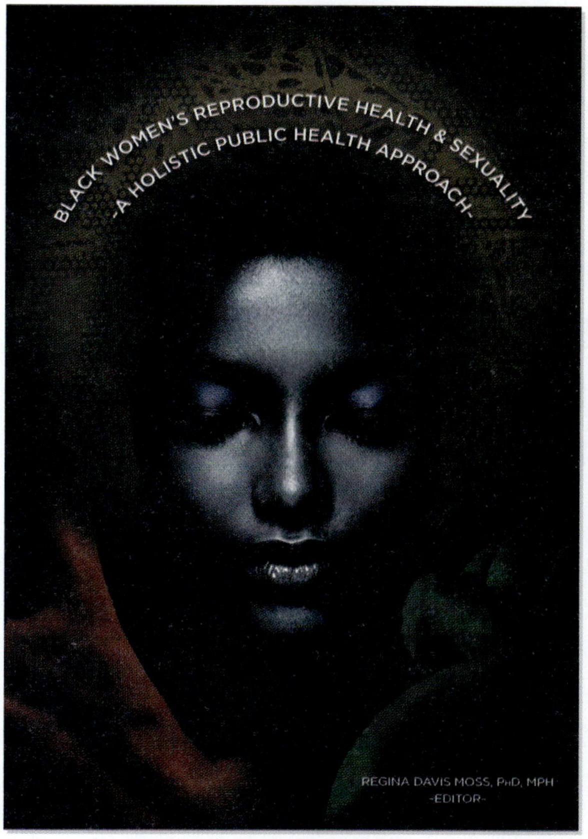

978-0-87553-340-7, 2023, 450 PP, SOFTCOVER

Black Women's Reproductive Health and Sexuality: A Holistic Public Health Approach

Edited by Regina Moss Davis, PhD, MPH

Reproductive health and sexual well-being are important parts of human health. But for Black women, research and education tend to focus on negative risks and outcomes. *Black Women's Reproductive Health and Sexuality: A Holistic Public Health Approach* offers a comprehensive look at the determinants of Black women's reproductive health and sexuality and shares evidence-based programs, policies, and promising solutions that support Black women in leading healthy and safe lives.

APHABOOKSTORE.ORG

APHA PRESS

AN IMPRINT OF **AMERICAN PUBLIC HEALTH ASSOCIATION**